WEIGHT LOSS WITH MINI HABITS

Change your Lifestyle

Without Dieting

Anna Patel

Disclaimer

The information contained in "WEIGHT LOSS WITH MINI HABITS" is meant to serve as a comprehensive collection of strategies that the author of this eBook has done research about. Summaries, strategies, tips and tricks are only recommendation by the author, and reading this eBook will not guarantee that one's results will exactly mirror the author's results. The author of the eBook has made all reasonable effort to provide current and accurate information for the readers of the eBook. The author and it's associates will not be held liable for any unintentional error or omissions that may be found. The material in the eBook may include information by third parties. Third party materials comprise of opinions expressed by their owners. As such, the author of the eBook does not assume responsibility or liability for any third party material or opinions. Whether because of the progression of the internet, or the unforeseen changes in company policy and editorial submission guidelines, what is stated as fact at the time of this writing may become autdated or inapplicable later.

The eBook is copyright © 2020 By Anna Patel with all rights reserved. It is illegal to redistribute , copy, or create derivative work from this eBook whole or in part. No parts of this report may be reproduced or retransmitted in any reproduced or retransmitted in any forms whatsoever without the writing expressed and signed permission from the author.

Table of Contents

INTRODUCTION 1

CHAPTER ONE: Healthy Weight Loss Habits 3

   Develop Successful Weight Loss Habits - Be Consistent ... 7

   Three Healthy Weight Loss Habits 10

CHAPTER TWO: Steps For Weight Loss 16

   The Effects Of Habits On Weight Loss 21

   Easy Weight Loss - A Weight off Your Mind 27

CHAPTER THREE: A Healthy Weight Loss Panel 34

   Weight Loss Through Hypnotism 41

   How to Reduce Back Pain and Sciatica - Weight Loss and the Buddy Plan 47

CHAPTER FOUR: Dos and Don'ts of Weight Loss 52

   Hypnosis Weight Loss - The Problems With Goal Setting 57

   Weight Loss - Why Hypnosis Really Does Help 62

CHAPTER FIVE: Weight Loss Without Diet 69

   Ease Into Your Diet For Stress Free Weight Loss Success 77

   Weight Loss - Tracking the Elusive Calorie 83

CHAPTER SIX: Lifestyle Changes Needed For Effective Weight Loss 88

Better Body Composition Or Simple Weight Loss? 94

Dieting is nothing In Losing Weight............................. 98

If Diets and Weight Loss Programs Leave You Cold - Start Your Own! 103

CHAPTER SEVEN: Weight Loss And Metabolism 109

Weight Loss and Your Health 116

A Simple Diet And Exercise Plan To Lose One Pound A Week.. 127

CONCLUSION... 137

INTRODUCTION

It is very apparent that most people consider weight loss as something related to their own personal suffering, as if each individual weight loss program required your sacrifice, to work effectively. When you think of issues such as poverty, desertion, doubt, and misery, you know exactly what I'm talking about; but for anyone, it shouldn't be the weight loss.

How do we develop a new pattern of weight loss? The development of new patterns has two main factors. The first is a repeat. We've only got to begin doing something! We were all very keen to set new goals and dream of what this task would bring to us, but it is just not enough excitement to realize our dreams. We have to enforce these strategies if we are to see any progress.

If you know it or not, you have probably developed food habits that interfere with your loss of weight. This makes this difficult to lose weight when your habits influence your behavior. Making radical changes at once might not be the best option because it is difficult for you to give up old habits. But it's a good idea to recognize your bad habits, so you can become mindful of them and work to overcome them and meet your weight loss goals.

CHAPTER ONE:
Healthy Weight Loss Habits

What are the best habit of weight loss for you to stay in the best form of your life? Staying in shape and preserving optimal health requires a well-balanced diet with low calories and fat. All that needs to be said is improved physical activity in combination with aerobic or cardiovascular exercises that increase strength, flexibility and movements. A good diet accommodates multifunctional food options and allows versatility in meal planning and exercise so that a person can stay fit even during stress or slight setbacks. Here are patterns of weight loss worth considering.

The best diet strategies to lose pounds and hold them off are those that fit with one's own lifestyle, food preferences, budget and schedule. For example, a Mediterranean diet is popular with many dieters primarily because it shows an abundance of entire foods (as opposed to processed foods) low in calories and bad fats. It is encouraged to eat vegetables-fresh green leafy kinds, roasted to perfecto or nuts, with a splash of extra virgin olive oil, herbs and spices. In addition, a flexible diet plan concentrates on consuming a huge portion of the food in lean protein sources, such as legumes or fish and whole grains. Dietitians are encouraged to drink plenty of water that supplements every meal.

MODIFY AND IMPROVE BEHAVIOR

A bad habit is the most basic, but most complicated of all weight loss habits. Eating only if you are hungry is a very important lesson, but it takes discipline so that you can stay in shape. During meals, a person is recommended for chewing food attentively and slowly and drinking plenty of water to avoid over-eating. To cure inevitable hunger between meals, it is recommended to eat small, healthy snacks. If a dietitian has a strong impulse to eat binge or to eat because of fear, depression or wrath, deep breathing and meditation are instead prescribed. Good exercises to fight unconscious food are yoga, walking and meditation.

HEALTHIER FOOD CHOICES

One of the best ways of bridging the gap between the amount of calories one absorbs and the quantity you eat is to replace wiser food. This can be achieved by beginning the day with a bowl of fiber-rich oats with fruit such as berries and bananas. The fiber allows a dieter to live longer while the flavor of the fruits tends to cure the sugar. Instead of having a low-carb lunch or dinner, sodium and calories would be better for whole grains and lean proteins that are low in fat. Many good full grain sources include brown rice, wild rice, whole wheat pasta, polenta, quinoa, couscous and wheat bread. Meat, fish, chicken and certain parts of beef are sources of lean protein. Extra virgin fats are sources of healthy fats, canola oil and avocados.

The other important element of the weight loss equation is the workout.

IMPROVED PHYSICAL ACTIVITY

When it comes to healthy weight loss, burning calories with physical activity or increasing physical activity is the right approach. Experts recommend that the average adult receive at least 30 minutes of physical activity four days a week to give way to weight loss. If someone stays inactive or does not raise their physical activity level, all other weight loss behaviors will be unhealthy.

Weight Loss Habit

We will implement weight loss habit #3 this week. Now you should keep your thoughts and behaviors in a positive direction and take your water where it needs to be for the optimal hydration of the body.

We're going to the third week now. Continue to implement the first 2 habits and add habit this week to your routine.

This week's routine of weight loss is an aerobic activity. The first thing I would like to do is explain the importance of aerobics.

Aerobic means essentially "with oxygen." Aerobic exercise requires oxygen in the metabolic processes that generate energy. It raises your metabolism, which uses energy for your fat storage.

Aerobic exercise is most commonly called a "cardio" workout. For starters, running is a "cardio" training. We increase the rate of heart and respiration. It strengthens both our cardiovascular system and our breathing system. In fact (better back, better lungs).

Without getting into numbers for ideal cardiac frequence areas, this is the fundamental principle for good training if you don't breathe hard and sweat.

Cardio should be done at least four days a week at a cat, at least 30 minutes a day. You should increase your days to 5-6 days per week if you live a very sedentary lifestyle. Here are some examples: -

Power walking-Jogging-

Jumping rope-Aerobics

Jumping Jacks

Develop Successful Weight Loss Habits - Be Consistent

Let's face it, consistency is not the most exciting characteristic, but all successful people do. He wasn't by mistake the most successful Formula 1 driver, Michael Schumacher has consistently worked hours and hours on the track to develop his skills. He didn't just spend a couple of laps on a Monday before he had the rest of the week off. The majority of high-performers attribute their success to hard work and to discipline, in other words to work diligently every day and never give up.

Most people go on a diet or start a weight loss program, only to finish up because they have not made success or obtained the desired results. In many cases, they were simply not sufficiently consistent and thus received the rewards they deserved. Healthy meals or daily workouts are not just things you do during the week (or if you like it) and forget all weekend. You need to be consistent in your efforts to lose weight to reap the benefits you want. But how can we build positive patterns of weight loss, including consistency?

Consistent with your attempts for weight loss, you do not all eat and do the same things day after day in robotic fashion. It is about being prepared, sensitive, controlled and healthy choices, and putting real effort and hard work into them. If you eat a balanced diet from Monday to Friday, but then blow out completely on the weekend, because you think you deserve a reward for all your hard work, it's not going to happen to you.

Let's look at how you can make the effort to lose weight more effective.

1. Prepare meals in advance Think about your next shop trip and buy fresher, healthier foods and unhealthy snacks. Plan your meals for the week ahead and encourage (in moderation) the occasional treatment meal. Keeping a healthy and well-designed food plan will give you more control over your daily consumption of calories.

2. Exercise Management One reason you are overweight is probably because you are eating. Begin to eat smaller, more responsive portions at each meal. If you match your serving size, you'll have a lot of calories cut from your diet. Your food should provide you with enough food, but not bloated or stuffed.

3. Take REGULAR exercise Consistency is the key to your success in practice. The only way you can

establish a good practice is by constantly performing consistently. At least 3 to 4 cardio exercise sessions a week, each consisting of at least 30 minutes. Even during rest days, become more active. Walk rather than use the car, take the stairs than the elevator and, instead of watching a movie, do something fun with the baby.

4. We're all human and there will be times when we're going to have a reversal. It's not important to have this odd slip, but what you learn and do afterwards. Just return as soon as possible to your healthy habits and do not use it for an excuse to give up.

The successful development of weight loss habits means consistency on a daily basis. If you can master consistency, your weight loss goals are reached

Three Healthy Weight Loss Habits

Pop quiz! Quiz! When is a roller coaster going to stop being fun? The answer? The answer? If it is your own nutritional roller coaster! We all did it—losing 10 pounds in one month, just to win 15. You tried Atkins, Jenny Craig, Weight Watchers, and nothing worked. Okay, I'm here to convince you that weight loss is a better way, and it's much simpler than you can imagine. The best way to permanently lose weight is simply to shape three simple safe customs.

But I want to address three basic principles before I expose these simple behaviors, which are necessary for a permanent change in your life.

Principle 1: If you want different results you have to do different actions

I think Albert Einstein said best, " The explanation of insanity always does the same thing and expects different results." When you think about it, it's a really insane thing to do using the same concepts which have failed you over and over to try and lose weight.

So, forget to get on the next major diet train. The best solution is typically the simple one most often ignored. If you think logically about it, short-term starvation can only lead to short-term weight loss. You may think that if you can only lose weight, you can adjust and keep your lifestyle off. One of the flaws in this plan is that you die so hungry that the diet is followed by a period of binge consumption that simply piles up the weight. The other thing is that you did not develop a new way to eat after a good diet, so you just fall back into your old habits. The consequence is that you lose a couple of pounds, and then you get those more. The bottom line is, remember what Einstein said before this time you started your weight loss program, and don't be insane.

Principle 2: You must choose.

Do you understand how much power you have to make choices about your body? You have to realize that you are not stuck in every loop, but that you have the freedom to choose your own path, regardless of your current circumstances. You can now choose to make changes that will help you lose weight, feel great, and enjoy higher living conditions.

Let us show this easily with two short questions: do you think that, over the coming weeks or months, you will be able to develop some new habit that will help you gain weight and improve your health?

Would you think that in a few weeks or months, you will develop new habits that would help you lose weight and improve your health?

The answer to both of these questions is, of course, yes! The true beauty of this case is that you have to pick 100%.

Principle 3: Above all, human beings are living things.

I'm sure that you heard this word before. Unfortunately, being habituated creatures means that we develop bad habits as quickly, easily, and sometimes as we develop good ones. Luckily, it is the maintenance of good living habits that is necessary to improve your health, work, and relationships.

"Motivation is what gets you are going, but only customs are what keeps you going." All right now, let's end up over those healthy customs that you want to develop: 1. Eat twice as much as normal.

This plan already looks better, isn't it? Well, don't be too excited to read the second habit. It is recommended for all chronic diseases to have five to six meals/snacks a day and is by far the best program for people who want to lose weight This helps to keep your metabolism working throughout the day, your blood sugar levels consistent and also prevents you from ever feeling hungry.

2. Just eat half, as usual, Our bodies tell us naturally when we are full. We just have to learn to hear. We feed well after we are finished several times simply because we have food on the plate. The best way to fight this is to put half the food on your table and eat it slower. Just developing this habit alone will surprise you how fully satisfied and fulfilled you are. When you eat out, just ask your server to put half of your order in a box, and then you can have it later. Then you can finish your plate as you have been taught and later.

3. Drink 6 to 8 glasses of water Every day, and more water is probably the toughest habit of forming... And one of the most important. Water seems just dull, with so many competing drinks to lure us. The human body comprises between 55 and 78 percent of the water at any time. Your body needs a certain water intake to

function and avoid dehydration. From many things, including food, we get water. Your body tells you to get more if you don't drink enough water. And if more water comes from food than from consuming it, the body is simply going to ask for food when it needs water.

Research from Washington University found that when people drank a glass of water during their meal when they were hungry, it fulfilled their hunger almost 100 percent of the time. You can also prevent the use of unwanted and unneeded beverage calories in your system by drinking more water.

Losing weight for life is not rocket science, but some basic, powerful habits are established. Develop the three simple customs above and get off the roller coaster for good!

CHAPTER TWO:
Steps For Weight Loss

You will finish a major project in two hours, so you go to the manufacturer for a high-calorie treat. With an important meeting just minutes away, you are stuck in traffic and start to bit your nails. You know that you should go to bed and sleep, but you can't look like you're turning off the TV. Would you know any of these scenarios? If so, you're stress-relieving bad habits.

Habits are repeated, probably unconscious behavior patterns. Everyone's got customs. Structure, stability, and safety are provided by positive habits. Good habits like good food, exercise, journaling, or talking to a friend, can alleviate tension. Negative habits can be self-destructive, and our self-esteem and self-worth can be negative. Bad habits often include stress-relieving or stress-relieving.

Unfortunately, in our lives, bad habits serve a purpose. These are risky methods for dealing with immediate benefits. The short-term gain involves stress reduction, a relaxation of our nerves, and a diversion or release from stressful circumstances or feelings. The long-term consequences include weight gain, unattractive nails, and tiredness. If your life is messed with by long-term effects, you will change your habits. You must find healthy coping strategies, which will pay you the short term.

Your realization and wish to change your way of life can be immediate. You decide that you are tired of a certain habit or conduct and are committed to replacing it. Alternatively, you may want to change your bad habits and need a gradual plan. If one of these is yours, it is time to continue replacing your habit.

Stage 1: Name it! Name it! Define the habit. Define habit. You must identify the reason for the habit before you can make any changes. What's the habit of paying you? Bad habits usually serve an unrecognized purpose. It can be used as a shield for tense feelings or even relaxed anxieties.

Step 2: Engage! Engage fully to change this habit. Inspire yourself to sustain motivation. Motivation has levels of motivation. Prepare for those days when there is low motivation, and you are tempted to go back to bad practice. Whatever motivates and inspires you, plan your reversal to use those tools when you need extra motivation to break the bad habit.

Step 3: Set short and long-term goals. Would you like to lose weight? Wanna lose 50 pounds? Split your goal of losing 50 pounds into small increments that you can reach. You don't want to get distracted. In just two months, you won't lose 50 pounds.

Step 4: Identify your triggers and remove them. Is some food a problem for you? Do you go directly to the kitchen to reach the comfort food to calm you from the day when you hit the work door? If so, don't have that in your house to cause food. Have healthy alternatives for snacks readily available. Instead, take the family and walk back home and talk. Set up the world to help you when you leave a bad habit.

Step 5: Get help. Ask your family and friends for the support that is important to you. Changing a bad habit is better if a support system is in place. If you want to lose weight, hiring a weight loss coach is a very effective way of helping. The help you need is offered by a weight loss coach. Your coach can help you create a personal program to help you change your habits to promote your objectives.

Step 6: You have to replace it with a positive one if you give up bad habits that have given you a payoff. A good habit, like eating otherwise to lose weight, exercise, or relaxation, can help you manage stress healthily. If you are going to eat late in the evening, replace it with a hobby like word riddles or counted cross-stitches to get your hands busy. It is important to replace bad habits with new, positive habits to maximize your success. The bad habit won't attract you anymore until you know it, and the good habits will be second nature and normal.

Step 7: Get rewards for yourself. If you lose 5 pounds, reward yourself. Reward yourself. Buy a magazine subscription for 10 pounds to support your new habit. Loan yourself with a new outfit or a pair of smaller jeans for a larger weight loss of 20 pounds. You certainly deserve one, since you are keeping to your goals and substituting a new, positive habit for bad habits. Recall that your reward reflects your goal. Reward yourself with non-food rewards for losing weight.

Step 8: Accept boards. Identify that plateaus are part of the process. Motivation is high when you begin to change your habits. When there are a plateau and nothing appears to be happening. You may even want to get back to the rewards that the bad habit gives. Nonetheless, plateaus are our way of adapting and get used to new positive behaviors. Your process will continue with possible adjustment plateaus. You can become frustrated during a plateau and want to stop because you don't make the progress you want. You will be able to continue with your target if you foresee it as part of the transition.

Step 9: Give yourself credit for your decision to change bad habits. Be kind to you. Be kind to you. A bad habit is not a judgment as a person regarding you. It means you have created a bad habit that no longer works for you. It's indicative that now you realize your ability to have a healthier, better, and happier life by replacing bad tradition. Recognize your own personal development.

Bad habits like excessive compulsive consumption have payoffs. Recognize how your life is constrained by bad habits. Follow these steps to make you feel better and improve behaviors so that your weight loss is accomplished and your weight loss target is maintained.

The Effects Of Habits On Weight Loss

Habits make your weight loss or ruin it. I will guide you through 10 positive habit-making steps. Start with the problem and the implementation of new and healthier behaviors.

1. Why build a habit

If we like it, our habits don't rule our life. These can be small things like brushing your teeth into large habits such as eating habits. Everywhere you look in your life, and you can see that habits are created and how you do stuff.

But don't let this frighten you. The good thing is new and good habits can always be formed. It ensures that your lives are dominated by your patterns. However, you control them. The problem lies in making these daily habits constructive and successful. Habits that take the loss of weight where you want it to go.

2. The process to make a habit.

The question now is how to make a habit. NASA conducted a study of sunglasses. There were some kinds of sunglasses. NASA wanted the astronauts to check. The only problem is that they messed with the vision of the astronauts. NASA decided to try them for an experiment. Over 30 days, the astronauts were wearing their sunglasses directly; they didn't take them off. After that period, they found that the eyes and minds of the astronauts had adjusted without problems for the use of those sunglasses.

The interesting part of the study is here. If an astronaut takes the goggles off for a day before the end of the 30 days, his body becomes human again. That astronaut should restart the 30-day count, and time was lost every day with the sunglasses.

Here is what it's all about habits. To make your life a habit, you have to make it straight for 30 days. It means you can't even stop your diet or exercise for 30 days. Like with the NASA report, if you take a break, you will restart to build this habit in your life.

3. What a custom in your life.

As I mentioned before, your life from small to big things controls your habits. Take food as an example. When you make a habit of eating healthy, you will want to eat good food instead of bad food. It is important to know that the best thing a tradition does in your life is to build an intense desire to do what you want.

4. Use of habit

The good news is that you can make habits work for you. The wrong thing is that habits can work against you. You need to think carefully and consciously about what patterns exist in your life. Tell yourself if the behaviors you manage are the ones you want to achieve your goals.

5. Habit Types:

Eliminating When you decide, you can possibly see habits you do not like, and go through the list of habits you have in your life. The first step of your life to remove the habit to know that the habit exists, and you want to remove it.

6. Habit Types:

Development The next step is to choose the habits in your life. Talk about what you want to do in your life. Which habits do you have to do? Make a list of the top 5 admirers. Write down the five habits you have in your life to lead you to the same success. I guess if I want to learn that the best option is to speak to the person and ask him what he thinks is important. By doing this, you might be shocked by what you know.

7. Swap Habits

You'll have to swap one habit with another to avoid one habit. They're like your life's roots. If you try to pull one out of your life, you'll have to replace another. Let's presume, for starters, that you've got a habit of drinking soda pop and have decided to leave. You have to replace it with something else, such as drinking water.

8. Start Small Habits

One problem many people experience is that they start to get big. For starters, let's take exercise. You want to make your life the habit of regular exercise. You go to the local gym and register to become a member. Then, three times a week, you decide to pump weights. The problem with this solution is that most people do not continue their training. It is because they concentrate on the wrong solution. Instead of developing a practice routine, they only begin to practice and then quit within a short time.

The right way to choose this workout target is to start doing a little training 15 minutes a day. Walking or riding a bike could be included. The goal with this, however, is to do it straight for 30 days, as we know this is going to create a habit. The tradition is part of you, and you want to practice every day. This is the strength of a habit.

9. Create Habits

Build one at a time your habits. Imagine creating a new habit every month of the year and replacing an old habit. I know that it's probably not as easy as you want things to change, but you're going to have 12 new habits at the end of the year. That's enough to change your entire life completely. Imagine what's going to happen over two, five, or ten years.

10. Always move forward with your habits.

It is always good to continue with your good habits. In physics, you learn that something gains momentum or loses momentum. There is never a time when stuff just stays where it is. You always have to analyze and change your ways of doing and moving forward. Make sure that you always evaluate and decide if you have a better habit of losing weight or improving your habit. You will always be responsible for your habits, which ensures that you control your life.

Easy Weight Loss - A Weight off Your Mind

Is there a long way to live?

I was surprised at a recent conversation as I put pen to paper (or fingers to keys) to write this chapter. The conversation was about diet, which always fascinates me because the majority of women I know are obsessed with eating and drinking due to their endless diet! My colleague stirred up about the many food plans that she pursued and how fantastic they seemed at first but eventually failed miserably. She sighed and seemed to be resigned to the endless battle of the life-long diet, a tough chore for anyone!

But before I could offer advice or support, my colleague piped up, hoping in her voice, "Perhaps I'm going to try this hypnosis." Now music was to my ears. As a qualified hypnotherapist, I am always surprised at how many people end up with hypnosis or hypnotherapy. You will have tried to overcome their problems of weight, smoking habits, phobia, and so on and turn to hypnotherapy when you have lost all hope that's your first error!

It's a well-known fact that more than 90% of diets fail and worse than that, after working so hard to lose weight, 30% of people lose weight, but all of them back on more! Diets may work in the short run, but weight gain is unavoidable once the old eating habits are restored. In order to successfully lose weight, unhealthy eating habits must be modified over the long term, and no diet will do that.

Furthermore, as people, we are driven by the principle of "pleasure and pain" and govern all aspects of our lives from the work we have chosen to spend our weekends. We're driven to look for pleasure (chocolate comfort or a glass of wine) and try to avoid pain (the arduous fight to eat what we really do not want and not eat what we like!). So we' try' with minimal effort to lose weight as we fear the struggle and pain that it will eventually cause us.

This is, of course, not the case for everyone. Some people have a positive and healthy way of eating, meaning that they eat what is right for their bodies and that knowledge makes them happy. Dain to them would be a diet full of fat and sugar, etc. And why do some of us struggle to eat healthily and to maintain an ideal weight every day, while others live with no idea of what a diet involves?

Emotions well play an important role in our food relation-the "comfort eater" (compulsive eater) will eat to maintain any negative emotions, regardless of whether they feel good enough or not. How many of you took comfort, literally in a glass of wine, some chocolate or other snacks, after a bad day in the office or with the children? And after relief, we experience' sorrow' or remorse when we've overgrown, causing us to find pleasure again in order to overcome this pain. And so the comfort eating cycle begins.

Many people simply have poor eating habits, which they acquired during their infancy or later in their lives. Unhealthy eating habits will, like any habit, be difficult to overcome and replace with healthier eating practices. Bad, unhealthy eating habits must be revamped and new, healthier ones improved, in order for people to lose/keep their body and weight safe.

So how can we eat comfort and food habits effectively, easily and naturally, and also sustain weight loss? Most diets (especially those that supplement actual meals) do not alter the individual's eating habits while working in the short term, and, as mentioned previously, once we stop eating, we go back to our old eating habits, which in the first instance caused our weight gain. There is, therefore, no surprise that the weight we struggled to lose slows down.

If you can permanently change your eating habits, there is no need for food or diet. So we see why certain dietary approaches do not encourage people to overcome their poor eating behavior, as it eventually affects their company and income! This is not the case for all diets however-some diet clubs are specifically designed to help us change our eating habits and provide support along the way so that we can eat healthily once and for everything and maintain an ideal weight.

So if you want to lose weight and keep it hidden, the only way is to change your eating habits. And how are you doing that?

You can use one of the many diet clubs that offer healthy dietary plans and advice on naturally, positively, and long-term weight loss. You learn to follow healthier eating habits as well as gain much needed support from the leaders and other participants, which is important, particularly in the first cycle, as you aim to alter what might be a lifelong habit.

You can take the journey yourself, relying on your will to be a healthier, slimmer, and fitter person. Make sure you get a lot of support from friends and families, and if you are a mother like myself, add new, healthier meals to the meal times of the family so that the entire family will benefit.

If you do not have the desire to change your diet and have tried and failed in the past, hypnotherapy is an excellent way to lose weight without losing your motivation easily. Hypnotherapy is a modern and popular form of weight loss that does not include a diet and does not involve the power of choice. So how does hypnotherapy work, and why is the loss of weight using this method so much easier than through diet?

Hypnotherapy enables compulsive and habit-eating people to lose weight successfully and effortlessly by reprogramming the unconscious mind into a healthy, positive diet. For the compulsory eater, however, it is important to first identify and address the cause of their diet before any improvements in their eating habits can be made. This over-catering duty usually comes from childhood / early adolescence and may be easy as a mixture of food as a reward when a child receives food for being successful or working hard in school.

For compulsive and habit eaters, weight loss can only be achieved by altering their eating habits. Hypnotherapy overrides their old negative eating habits and substitutes them for better healthy eating habits. Habits are embedded in the unconscious mind and fall into the background unconsciously without us understanding them. So, to alter our eating habits permanently, this change must occur in the depths of our mind-the unconscious mind. Hypnotherapy allows us to connect with the unconscious mind, to erase current eating patterns, and to substitute them with constructive, healthy eating behavior.

After our unconscious mind has rooted in these new eating patterns, our fight against diet comes to an end. We have chosen healthy food and smaller portions consciously and feel less willing to eat between meals because we feel comfortable after each meal.

Whether large portions, succulent foods, snacking, etc. hypnotherapy can thus help you to conquer and substitute it with more healthy habits, which encourage you to lose too much weight and sustain the weight loss.

If you have suffered from a long diet for years, then hypnotherapy is for you. Hypnotherapy is a fast and easy way to lose weight as opposed to the years of battling the bulge, which usually takes six sessions. In addition, eating a healthy balanced diet can not only help you lose weight but also contribute to overall health and vitality, together with confidence. It can even help to improve the mood.

Then think twice next time you see what diets are available on the web. Would you like long-term or short-term gains?

CHAPTER THREE:
A Healthy Weight Loss Panel

Not all people have been made equal. Some are short, and others are tall, eye color, hair color, and skin tones vary. These are things that are beyond our control. This is how we were born, and we can always point our finger at our genetic makeup when we end up dissatisfied because of how we look.

But there are several things we can do in order to present ourselves more clearly to the rest of the "people" and achieve the feeling and trust we get when we know that we look good. Hairstyles, grooming, personal care, and the way we dress all relate to our look. And, of course, how much do we weigh on the one question which preys on all our minds?

The multitude of available choices makes it hard to find out which is the best, or even if weight loss plans work at all? They function on a fundamental level. Each of them will help you to lose weight. But shouldn't a stable, sustained weight loss really be the goal?

Most people tend to notice progress immediately when they plan. You find a weight loss plan, follow it, start weight loss, and feel good about yourself. Instead, they lose focus and e-daisy! The obese marches like a proud hero and destroys all the hard work.

If you are really preparing to become slimmer, a long-term commitment to the mission is important. You have to go out and find your soul mate, the most appropriate weight loss plan. And then you're running it, knowing it. Once you have compatibility, you agree to marry the weight loss plan and make it part of your life.

Should I even lose weight?

You should stop and ask yourselves some questions first before you put on your armor and head out into the battlefield for a cruise against high body fat. Were you actually overweight or not? How much weight must you lose? People begin on this path, and occasionally they forget to look back. They forget that it is most important to remain healthy, not the numbers on the weighing machine.

Why do you first want to lose weight? Is your health worries disturbing, or vanity? Is it, maybe, a bruised ego-comments at work or a social gathering? It is a long dark road leading to a lean, healthy body. You need the right motivation to travel and overcome barriers on the way. Do not let opinions of other people cloud your judgment and surrender halfway, for the timid will remain fat forever!

How do I go about weight loss?

Well, it's really pretty simple. You're hungry. No? No? But you're going to lose weight!

But that's not really the goal, is it? It ought not to be. Weight loss alone should never be the target, because hunger will do this to you, and it's simple. No, the objective is to develop and maintain a good-looking, healthy body. Above all, a body that makes you feel good.

You should now have been talking about why you want to or need to lose weight, how much you need to lose, and how much you want to lose.

Now that you're all set and inspired to start the slim program let's talk about the various approaches and techniques which can help you lose weight. Essentially, there are only three ways: eating plans, workout routines, or a mix of diet and exercise.

Most people don't need a weight loss plan. We only need to change a few daily habits marginally, and they will see the changes they expected. Sometimes the only obstacles that are in our way are our daily activities or our eating habits.

It is not only important to eat well, but also crucial to eat properly, which most people don't realize. The same theory is also applicable to sleep. The perfect time to sleep is 10:00 p.m. Six hours at night until 04:00 a.m. In the morning. In the morning.

Then plan your meals and sleep patterns, plan the rest of your day and then stick to the schedule. You will find almost noticeable changes in your body and overall health.

However, most people need a proper weight loss plan. Just fixing your eating or sleeping habits won't make the necessary changes. Some of them are too busy or too lazy to do any activity in their daily lives and need dietary plans only. Many love to eat so much, they want a workout schedule only, so they don't have to compromise nutritionally. Some others opt for the full fitness package and recommend a healthy weight loss plan that includes both exercise and a healthy diet.

As described in the previous chapter, often, everything that is required to lose the few extra pounds of fat is a minor alteration in our daily habits.

The excess weight that you desperately try to get rid of with complex diet and workout programs can only be the result of habits that are not even in your food patterns.

1. Tricks n' tricks. Wake! Sleep! There can be little focus on the importance of good, long, and easy sleep at the right time. Lack of sleep can lead to excessive eating, and therefore weight issues, by stimulating appetite.

2. It's cliché, but breakfast is the biggest meal of the day. This helps you to concentrate and provides the physical and mental strength to boost your metabolism for the rest of the day.

3. Preparation is all. Put the paper and stylus out and write down what you expect to eat for the week. Make a table, list the 21 meals, and then try your best to adhere to the schedule.

4. The brain takes about 20 minutes to know that you should stop eating now. Tedious, eh? Tedious? Take time, slowly feed, and thoroughly chew. After all, there's really no rush.

5. Do your own shopping. Do your own cooking. Not only do you encourage yourself to play with a variety of food and tastes, but it can also be an entirely satisfying and enjoyable experience while helping you resist the urge to fatten junk food.

6. These are the spices that make one's life varied. Try new ones. Try new ones. People find dieting difficult

because they often confine themselves, including raw vegetables, too bland food. Spices don't fatten. Experiment with them to add new tastes to your cooking and make your diet more appealing to you.

7. Probably the most difficult advice to follow. Raid your fridge; take all that could put your diet plan off and get rid of it. Indeed, even if the cheese and the chocolates are included. Hey, and all the soft drinks!

8. Water sustains life, nurture life. Water sustains life. It is life. It is life. Drink at least one glass of water before each meal to keep your appetite under control and ensure that you drink eight or more water glasses every day.

9. Snacking is not good. Snacking is not pleasant. Get used to brushing your teeth after all you eat, and you're not tempted to eat as many or as often.

10. Stay active! Stay active! Find alternatives to some of the jobs. Go to the supermarket for food rather than driving. Take the steps to work rather than the lift.

Small, small changes like these can go a long way to help you lose weight and then maintain the weight loss.

Weight Loss Through Hypnotism

Hypnosis is an option for weight loss considered. It is a process by which your consciousness is temporarily altered. It is a type of psychotherapy that lets your conscious mind relax while your subconscious mind is open to suggestions or behavioral changes. It's normal and healthy.

Hypnotic treatment Some problems are considered to be a useful tool in addressing a number of issues- ulcers, anxiety, sexual dysfunction, sleep disorders, Reynaud's disease, pain, high blood pressure, learning disabilities, skin disorders, loss of weight, Crohn's disease, depression, concentration problems, allergies, asthma, stress management.

In your conscious mind,

Desires, desires, and needs are created. Your conduct is created on your subconscious level. You hear everything that is happening around you-the background noise and people talking when you are hypnotized. It is estimated that your subconscious mind is 88 percent more alert during hypnosis.

If you're hypnotized, your conscious mind is circumvented to make directions to your subconscious mind. Your unconscious mind will take these suggestions and create changes in your behavior or body in order to make the suggestions. In order to be the most effective way to lose weight, your hypnotist needs to understand your weight gain behavior before you start. Make sure the hypnotist knows what, how, and why you have gained in weight and what you have done in the past to lose weight. In order to help you in this process, you must first plan.

Personal preparation

You must believe it works absolutely-faith. Up to 15% of the population of the United States can be quickly hypnotized. Likewise, up to 15% of the population cannot be hypnotized. In fact, 85% of the population can be hypnotized. When you avoid hypnosis, it is quite possible that you will be hypnotized.

You have to have a sincere desire to work. It allows the subconscious to consider suggestions for weight loss better. You have to expect it to work as well. Expectancy drives the subconscious mind to act. Wishes and wishes remain in your conscious mind and do not affect your subconscious mind for a long time.

Brain Activity Levels

There are four stages of brain activity-Beta, Alpha, Theta, and Delta. When you are fully aware, you are at the beta level. If you're in a deep sleep, you're in the Delta. The level of alpha is just under consciousness, and the level of the Theta is just above deep sleep. You must be at the alpha level to be effective in hypnosis.

Most people experience brain activity at an alpha level many times a day. If you dream, you're at the level of the Omega. You are at Alpha point when you drive a car on' autopilot'–you arrive at your exit, and you cannot remember going past familiar landmarks on the road home. All around you can see and hear-just as in hypnosis.

Habits

Behaviors Hypnosis is a method for changing habits. You may have good habits, such as the right exercise and the right food. You may have bad habits like smoking or overeating. The subconscious does not determine the difference between good and bad habits or recognize it. It works out what you gave it over time. It takes 21-30 days to break a habit. This is why.

Portion Control

One powerful way to lose weight with hypnosis is' portional control.' You can eat out of politics because it is time for food, you are told not to leave food on your plate, you may not want to waste food — portion Control No matter why a pattern has been developed that is difficult to change. Hypnosis is highly effective for changing behavior in these situations, leading to weight loss.

Brain Body Balance

The ideas given during hypnosis go straight to your subconscious mind. Brain-Body Balance You want to keep your unconscious mind in contact with your body and its needs. Train them properly, and they'll know when they're finished and tell you to stop feeding. If you properly use portion control, food waste is reduced to a minimum.

Pictures and Visual Cues

Hypnotic recommendations on visual issues and photos are not directed at over-alimentation. The subconscious uses more visual signals and symbols than words. The word "over-reacting" is usually not used, because your subconscious can not process a good visual image. Rather, the term ' excess sludge' can be used to evoke a picture in your mind in order to see the effect you don't want. If you are eating too much, you place extra sludge in your bloodstream, and it pounds your body and makes it lenient.

In reality, you do not hear the term ' excessive sludge' because it has been planted or implied in your subconscious to' see' what actions you need to change or what behavior. You still have the same quality and quantity choices, but now you can only take one cookie, not three or more.

Temporary transition to lifelong progress

The prior views and attitudes regarding the ability to lose weight have been removed over time. It seems hopeless to try another diet because you all failed. Each time you try to change your behavior, your subconscious gets the mental tug of war. You could make small gains, but your success is usually short-lasting. Permanent change allows the subconscious to be re-programmed.

Self-hypnosis

So, can I do it myself if I need re-programming? The reply is YES. Equally effective and relatively easy is self-hypnosis. CDs, DVDs, videos, books, etc. are available from a variety of well-known sources. Be very careful about the goods you want your money and time to spend. For your investment, you want value.

One suggestion to use CDs before going to sleep. Normally this is a good time to offer suggestions to your unconscious mentality, but if the end of the CD tells you to wake up and feel' alert and refreshed,' that isn't the message when you get ready for sleep that you want to tell your brain.

How to Reduce Back Pain and Sciatica - Weight Loss and the Buddy Plan

Lower back pain is a condition that many people experience throughout their lives. New evidence suggests that being overweight or obese could cause many of the lower back pain suffered by people today, especially people who are too heavy or obese. A precise diagnosis of the cause of the pain is vital because back pain can have a myriad of causes and consequences.

Obesity has today become America's number one preventable disease. The higher the weight of a person, i.e., the stomach, "love handles," and the lower back, the higher the risk of low back pain and science.

Weight loss certainly reduces the discomfort and can potentially eliminate it entirely.

Programs for weight loss are not created equal. Every individual has a different metabolism, and what works for one pain and sciatic pain cannot work for another person. All of the key factors for a successful weight loss and back pain management strategy are, however, attitude, lifestyle changes, and motivation.

Attitude is crucial! Attitude is crucial! It's important to think that you can control the situation and your life. While the slogan "Yes I Can, Yes I Will" may seem to be just what the doctor ordered! Yeah, you will lose weight, yeah you lose weight! Yes, you lose weight. Start your weight loss program and keep thinking, "Oh, oh, yes, I will!" every day, think and practice it, retrain your brain, and program it with your positive attitude. The workout then brings you to a shift in your lifestyle, 17 days, and a routine becomes a pattern, your habits change.

Change in lifestyle will gradually come over time. It's hard to break old habits, and it doesn't always succeed if you take a "crash" strategy. Therefore, what often happens is a turnaround, a turn back to our old ways. If we want to change Rome overnight, we might actually go too quickly and fail in our enthusiasm. Start with a list of things you want to improve in your life, techniques to deal with your back pain, and sciatica effectively. You can find excuses not to walk a day. Put it at the top of the list! We all know that exercise is important for weight loss and is crucial as a strategy for back pain and sciatica. So look at what kind of food and snacks you carry in your house regularly. Do they help your weight and, therefore, your back pain and sciatica? Do you order high-fat foods such as French fries instead of salad when you eat out?

Goals in all weight loss and bad back approaches are also relevant. Start slowly and take only small steps to get there. "Baby steps out the door! Baby steps around the block!" After all, we built our lives, and one shouldn't have to change these habits overnight, they just don't work. Nonetheless, it may take time and effort to improve bad habits, but that can and should be achieved. Remember: "Yes, I will. Yes, I will." You're still being inspired. You will have motivation, successes and weight loss failures, and good days and bad days with your back pain. One of the greatest motivators, of course, was to see the scale decrease, and again to fit in that dress or these shorts, which were both in the dust collection cabinet. Weight loss is a great driver, weight loss, and a substantial reduction in the number of pain allows you to hit the block for extra time!

Rewards are extremely important as an integral part of any motivation plan. Change is hard, and if you have made some changes, progress your bad habits, give yourself a treat, go out in the city for a night... or just a split banana! This won't hurt; it will just continue to keep you and search for the next reward. Start planning not only your motivational technique, your back pain, and the sciatica prevention strategy, but also your incentive for working towards a certain target. As the old saying goes, we are all lazy creatures.

Don't be frustrated if the loss of weight isn't as fast as you want if you have bad back pain or sciatica episode. Remember to stay on track, concentrate on your goals, and achieve the results to which you are working. Don't go back; go ahead and remember: "Yes, I Can Yes I Will." Often it's good to use a buddy system, another person who also tries to achieve a target. You don't have to match your buddy's goals. The goals could be quite different from the one you try to achieve, that's okay. The most important component of a buddy system is that you know each other's goals and are fully committed to helping the other person, your friend, reach their goals. Are there others in your household, or have you a friend who should lose weight? Does anybody you know have back pain and/or sciatica and a few too many pounds? Say that both of you work together to achieve your goals. It will help both of you and help you to stay motivated and on track. Ideally, you will be both less weighty, weight loss targets met, and back pain and sciatica reduced or eliminated dramatically!

A successful strategy for weight loss starts with a strong foundation of mindset, lifestyle, and motivation. Harmony of purposes and selfless alliance are key components that enable back pain and sciatica patients with too much weight to balance their lifestyles, to eliminate bad habits, to succeed in their weight loss scheme, and to reduce back pain and sciatica by a partnership and effective bad back strategy!

CHAPTER FOUR:
Dos and Don'ts of Weight Loss

Here are 5 DO and NO weight losses to be concentrated on if weight loss and better shape are a top priority. The hardest part of this is consistency, but the more frequently you keep to the process, the faster you develop healthier living habits to lead you through every day. Here are the 5 DOs of loss of weight: DO Drink plenty of water. This is one of the healthiest habits that you can start making every day. Replace soda, energy drink, or 0 calorie water for Gatorade. Water not only does nothing to add to your total daily calories, but it also helps to absorb and to eliminate impurities from the body. Try drinking water with every meal and consider 6-8 glasses a day.

DO Eat Adequate portion sizes

This is often the most overlooked aspect of the cycle of weight loss. Eating a suitable portion will help to ensure that you don't eat more than your body needs. If you eat to the extent that you're stuffed, you ate too much. Serve a suitable portion on your plate and eat slowly to allow your body to record the amount you enter. Combine a big glass of water with your proper serving size, and you will eat much less than you used to.

DO Cook For Yourself

If you've always known the fast food drive, or if you know the first name of the pizza deliverer, it's time to make some changes. Healthy food starts in your kitchen, so don't be afraid of your stove, oven, or fridge. They are your best allies when they are used properly. Find and try recipes that seem attractive to you. You can soon see why it's a great healthy practice to start cooking as often as you can.

The advantage of preparing yourself is that you can eat a little more deliberately so that you will have the leftovers to take with you to work the next day. Even if you're not working, the next day, you can still eat the remains that save you from cooking something. So, in essence, you may have prepared enough for two or even three meals if you cook a meal.

DO exercise 3-5 days per week

One of the best ways to burn the body's calories is through preparation. You will start looking forward to your time when you build this healthy habit. It may be completely alien to you right now, but once you have passed the two-month barrier, if you like the workouts that you choose, you will really come to take a break. Find a sport/activity you like to do, or you can even learn something from an instructor that you wanted to learn. Take it slowly but try and stick to these important DOs as best as possible and you will lose weight week after week consistently. Keep in mind that, even losing a pound a week, in just a year, you will lose 52 pounds. You want 50 + pounds lighter from now on a year?

Now for 5 DON'Ts of the weight loss process. Try to avoid doing these things as you work to create and maintain healthy living habits.

DON'T Overeat

Overeating is hand-tied to portion size. Often, we lose our conversation during meals or look distracted on the TV and can easily overlook how much food we put on our bodies. Healthy eating habits would mean eating a good serving size, drinking lots of water, and going on. Don't get too packed to the point where the damage is done by then, and it's too late. In other words, you should not get stuffed to release your grip on the fork and knife.

If you've stopped tracking the nutritional content of your favorite fast-food meals, then you'll be shocked to know that total calories can go beyond 2,000 points. Sadly this is more than enough calories for a whole day in many fast foods! Don't pack your body that much food at once. This is one more explanation of why it is so important that you start to cook regularly AND serve appropriate portion sizes for those meals.

DON'T Eat Late At night

Your body won't do any good if you eat a great meal before bed. Try not to eat less than 3 hours before you go to bed. You must give your body time to consume some of the food that is not going to happen if you sleep shortly after eating.

Do not eat / snack while watching TV

For any other things, including reading a book or using the phone. Do not eat / snack. In moments like this, our mind is concerned, and our mouth and hand are moved automatically. Anyone who did this before was likely to see an empty box of cookies or potato chips 30 minutes later, asking where they were all going. Snacks of this type are extremely harmful to a healthy life.

DON'T Starve Yourself

For those who say they can lose more weight by starving their bodies, and they are totally wrong. Your body needs fuel every day in the form of food. Many people think that a day or two of hunger will help them lose a bunch of weight, but this is hardly the case. Usually, after the hunger period is over, the person is so hungry that he starts to overfish, clamping everything into his or her body. Since the body can not use all the food at once, the rest will only be added to your fat storage. Don't cause your body this needless pain. Feed your body good, well-served food, and you'll never have to pine for weight loss.

Hypnosis Weight Loss - The Problems With Goal Setting

You read it because you're overweight. Afterward, you tried to lose weight. You probably tried many times to lose weight. You wondered why others could lose weight so easily and keep it away permanently. Why can't you? Why can't you do that?

You can certainly fight and fight for the rest of your life to maintain your weight. You will forever jump to another fast weight loss diet, always looking for the best miracle weight loss pills or the next best weight loss program.

You can try these things... but they won't work for you!

You will never have that lean, slim body you want until you know first how to regulate your subconscious mind, change your subconscious mind, and use your subconscious power to think like a slim and tiny human.

When forming your convictions, feelings, and ideas, the subconscious mind is important. This is what your behavior and actions are all about. You have to change your beliefs, emotions, and thoughts to change your behavior and actions. You need to change your subconscious mind in order to change your values, feelings, and ideas.

To be a slim, thin person, you must first decide to be thin and slim. Did you choose to be thin and lean? If so, and you are still struggling to do so, there can be only one explanation. You have made a conscious decision to become lean and thin but have not decided to do so unconsciously. To be thin and lean at all times, you have to react, think, and act like a thin and slim person. You haven't yet been able to.

You probably set a goal to be thin and lean in the past. You were motivated, developed a plan, and began to act. But you worked every step of the way and fought to stay on your course and to keep you motivated. To make things worse, you had no idea why this was going on. Why was it all so hard?

The whole problem came from the "goal" setting process. Objectives have a clear attitude attached to them, "get there quickly." The act of setting goals can make you think so distracted about your future moment of achievement, that you lose full contact with the present and all actions that must continuously be taken to reach your moment of success.

Your ambitions will begin to feel more like work than anything else. No one wants to do things! Setting targets can also be frightening.

Sometimes, once you set a target, you feel "locked-in" and can't stop or give up because then you are a "failure" or a "quitter."

Why would someone want to fight and fight to accomplish anything while constantly dealing with a fear of failure to just hit a potential goal as quickly as possible? Of course, you will begin to question the whole thing first of all, wouldn't you? It's obvious that when someone starts to doubt the motivations for an action plan, they begin to lose the momentum and the enthusiasm they have started first of all. We know that inspiration and anticipation are two very important factors to accomplish something.

Why does setting the target lead to this?

This is because our goals are formed and derive energy from our CONSCIOUS MIND. This is the moral, logical part of us which "displays things out" and seeks "reasons" for doing things. The greatest difficulty in using your mind to set goals is that your conscious mind relies heavily on the power of the will to make things happen. You can force yourself to set targets, create action plans, and then try hard to keep them with your will. This is doomed to fail, however.

The reason this won't work is that you're upstream swimming. You fight AGAINST behavior and habits in your own lifetime.

Your brain has been learning how to do things in a certain way for many years. You have rituals, habits, and routines every day. Most of your behavior and actions are predetermined and monitor where your life goes. Then, you come along, set an agenda, and expect everything to change and change forever. Sorry, but this is not the way it works. There is only one way to change your life permanently. Your actions, behaviors, and acts are regulated by your unconscious mind's values, feelings, and emotions. If your beliefs, thoughts, and emotions can be changed, your behavior will change. If you can change your values, thoughts, and emotions in order to match and endorse the goals you want to achieve, your daily lives, attitudes, and behavior. Without having to fight or dealing with any feelings of failure and doubt, you will easily and quickly move to your "goals." You will never be able to use any weight loss diet plan, make and continue new healthy eating habits or build a new, slim, and lean lifestyle.

Everything will be AUTOMATICAL forever. Hypnotherapy and hypnosis are well known to be some of the most effective tools for accessing and manipulating the subconscious mind. These approaches and techniques are strong and proven. Many have been successfully tested and used by any society worldwide for decades! There are already legions of people with weight loss hypnosis for a safe loss of weight, normal loss of weight, rapid weight loss, and permanent weight loss. If so, many others use hypnosis effectively for weight loss, then you can! Make your decision, choose the best weight loss hypnotherapy, and the best weight loss diet for you and start weight loss today. You can do that! You can do it!

Weight Loss - Why Hypnosis Really Does Help

If you are one of the many millions of people who strive to maintain the right weight, you will probably know the generally accepted weight management principles. The rules say that you only need two things to maintain the right weight: diet and workout. Both aspects are explained in books and services in a trillion-dollar company worldwide.

Sadly, it fails, at least to make a difference, if not to make money for its directors. The proportion of overweight and indeed obese population is growing at an alarming rate. And by the way, it's not just the US. Global obesity is so serious that the World Health Organization has coined a new word "globesity," to describe what they consider to be a global problem.

For many of us, "proper diet and practice" is not a simple or easy answer, but a total and challenging change in lifestyles. Resistance to the necessary changes in personal eating and exercise practices is what many individual attempts to lose weight do.

In other words, proper diet and exercise is only half of what is needed to keep your weight healthy–physical half. This is the other half, which keeps us overweight: mental and emotional challenges, resistance to change, and difficulties breaking habits and routines.

And since "proper diet and exercise" is quite easy in principle, and the mental and behavioral problems are the benchmark, these last problems we will focus on. Hypnosis can help here.

By the way, I can comment that all this is why programs such as Jenny Craig, weight watchmakers, and even overheaters are so effective. Anonymous. They address your emotional needs as well as the physical aspects of diet through meetings and consultants to allow you to interact with others. The use of hypnosis can, however, be much cheaper, quicker, and easier.

For example, most of us are (conditioned) used to eating certain types and amounts of food on a specific schedule. It's not easy or different to eat. Our tummy is used to feeling full, our brains are conditioned at times to eat, and we are used to certain foods, often "not good" for us.

Exercise is not so easy to work into your daily routine, too. It seems simple, but people are resistant to it. Plus, who has the time in today's society?

Hypnotic techniques can help here. Hypnotherapy is about repairing patterns and improving behavior. A course of hypnotherapy can help you change your current behavior and habits, that is to say, the mental and emotional challenges, to adapt more easily to the new lifestyle necessary to achieve the two physical cornerstones of weight control diet and exercise.

Yet, hypnosis or not, you still have to eat and exercise. Hypnosis helps you do this. This helps you.

Now the good news is that a good hypnotherapy program can influence good behavior in weight management considerably and make a significant difference to the adaptations needed for a new diet and exercise regime.

First, you can learn relaxation from hypnosis. Many of the triggering factors that cause people to eat too much are caused by stress. The relaxation learned through hypnosis techniques can reduce stress significantly, making it much easier to adjust to new habits.

A good hypnotherapist will then work with you to detect triggers. Triggers are things in the environment that "causes" you to eat consciously or unconsciously at the wrong time. Drives good diet and exercise habits into sabotage.

You may be one of those who stand in the refrigerator for no reason and just seek something to eat. Your hypnotherapist will help you change your behaviors, so you can snack only at certain times and then only eat something good for you, for example, a protein snack to prevent hypoglycemia or low blood sugars.

Some foods are described as comforts-food that is delicious to eat and fill, and typically bad for you. For some people, comfort food is their whole diet. Perhaps their parents were fed comfort food when they were upset at a young age. Regardless of the reason, bad eating habits are now well established. Your hypnotherapist can suggest that you change automatic responses when you have a "stress moment" or an upset.

Hypnosis can actually contribute to alleviating the pangs or cravings that we tend to feel, even though we are not hungry and do not need food. We often eat because we are used to eating at some time, or because our stomachs feel comfortable. The problem is that over the years, we have to eat more and more to keep that feeling "full." Hypnosis will counteract this tendency to let go of the hunger pangs in the wrong times.

You can also help your hypnotherapist to change your mental patterns to make you feel better. Self-image is a major issue in terms of weight and diet.

Dieting, as it happens, is not difficult. There are a wide variety of options for people who want larger portions, people who like foods, and so on. It makes the adjustment that makes the difference to adhere to a plan, which is the key to success.

So, what's the plan for the game? First, it is always a good idea to visit your doctor and get advice on what to do and the limits when you get into any form of diet, exercise, or other changes in lifestyle. For instance, if you haven't exercised forever and you're overweight of 50 pounds, it's not a good idea to try 3 miles a day. You must begin slowly. Get your doctor's diet and exercise plan.

Next, understand, you must slowly take it. Weight loss of 1-2 pounds a week is a standard goal, and both diet and exercise are required. In the short term, you can probably lose more by taking more extreme measures like dieting from starvation. This does not last, however, and is not recommended.

Secondly, understand that even with hypnosis, you must exercise a little will. Hypnosis will greatly help you to understand the urges and reframe your automatic responses. However, you will have to say "no" at some point. At this point, a hypnotic refresher, like an MP3 record, is very effective.

Many "weight loss hypnosis" programs and CDs are available. However, the best type of program offers individual personalized sessions, backed up by recordings between the sessions. For example, Hypno-To-Go provides such a program. The individual hypnotherapy sessions that can be conducted over the phone will be directed to your particular weight loss problems and also be adapted to support the specific diet and exercise program you have chosen or recommended by your doctor.

Finally, you know you're not alone. Millions of people are overweight and even obese. This doesn't mean, however, that you can't change yourself. Take the right steps, take them slowly, and commit to the long run, and your future will certainly be a return to a lower standard. I wish you every success in your efforts to lose weight.

CHAPTER FIVE:
Weight Loss Without Diet

So, from the viewpoint of a layperson, I dare say that diets just make you fat.

There are, of course, exceptions: if you're super-rich and can afford your own personal chef or caterer, and you might not be protected by this rule. But, for the average person after a diet, it is too restrictive to survive for a long time. Who wants to weigh every bit before eating? Who wants to eat what a diet tells you exactly? A diet leaves no room for pressures or hunger or appetite, so a diet gives us a constant sensation of unhappiness and retention.

I firmly feel that a slim body can only be a satisfied, well-nourished body. Our bodies express in cravings their needs. When the idea of strawberry water my mouth, I guess my body needs a strawberry, and only a strawberry will satisfy me to the full extent that I feel comfortable.

Your body gets used to low-calorie intakes when you follow a diet. Once you get back to normal, your body loads happily on the pounds, and the effort is wasted. For all kinds of fasting or crash diet, this is especially true: once, she fasted absolutely for three weeks and lost her weight. However, my slim body lasted only one week. When she started eating again, my body sprang on all the calories it was denied — a very frustrating experience, not to mention the exhausting mental fight for three weeks to abstain.

According to my knowledge, you have to understand the reason why your body looks like it before losing any extra pounds.

Overweight reasons: There are a lot of reasons, but she dares say: most of the excess pounds we carry are rooted in our psyche. We tend to pile on the pounds when we take life too heavy. Are you too dependent on your shoulders? Do you really like to do more than you could? Or do you not realize that you suffer from depression?

If we really want our weight to shift, we need to look inward. Perhaps you've just too enjoyed the culinary pleasures of life and thus put extra pounds on. On the other hand, why do you need food or drink to comfort yourself?

It may now sound like pseudo-psychology, but a close person experiences it, and I know what I am talking about. If you have been dealing with your weight seriously for many years (no matter if you are overweight or not), you can look for help from a qualified psychotherapist or be offered psychological help in any way. A friend's sympathetic ear can not be overlooked.

Only if you find out what makes you fat can you lose weight?

I think one of the biggest reasons to pile up the pounds is the abundant amounts of chemicals mixed in modern food. First of all, there are different glucose and malt syrups, from your mouth directly into your blood and hips there.

Then there are all the preservatives in the digestive system that cause havoc. Think of the essence of a preservative: its purpose is to prevent bacteria from spoiling food. Sadly, our digestive system also works with the aid of bacteria. She can not imagine that food swamped with preservatives can easily be digested or can supply our body with enough nutrients.

If you like too much to eat, you eat a lot of unhealthy fats. Have you ever looked at the type of oil that a restaurant kitchen uses? She dares say anybody who wants to remain healthy should not drink fast food or restaurant on a daily basis.

The undetected yeast infection of the digestive system may also lead to overweight. Yeast infections are now widely spread and can be easily caught in any public place. They're very hard to get rid of. Candida albicans enter the digestive tract and consume the food we eat. As a result, food cravings and binge eat frequently.

How to stay slim or lose weight: after this has been written, let me show you how a lady has a dietless weight and a desire to eat and drink. For all of those that say they have foods that make you slim, she wants to say (it is obviously hard to get the weight to eat only leafy vegetables or green beans but who wants to live that way?): Only foods that don't enter your mouth don't make you fat.

Reduce the portions you eat if you want to lose weight, but don't deny anything to yourself. Give your appetite and your cravings, whether it's a chocolate pie or a French fries. Don't eat too much of the delights of sin. Stop following a little piece of cakes or a few French fries. Our bellies are habitual creatures: when used to smaller portions, you will feel satisfied with less. Permanent loss of weight is always a slow process, so you should be willing to eat less for a long time.

1. Move. Exercise. When people ask me how they get to stay slim over the years, they answer: they don't eat too much and go to the fitness center at least three times a week. There is no option for exercise at all. Our bodies have to function well. Exercise increases the heart rate, bringing more blood and nutrition to our cells. Exercise increases our metabolism and hormone production. You feel good and relaxed after a good

workout. It doesn't matter what workout you do; it's important to move your body and to pump your heart. She never thought of me as a sportsman, but after that, she likes to sweat in the gym because she feels so good. Fortunately, exercise is very addictive: after a training session, you start to feel great and enjoy it.

2. The beauty of love is the best way to lose weight. If we usually fall in love, we lose a few kilograms without even warning. Unfortunately, it is not possible to program this way of losing weight, although you can fall in love with yourself. When was the last time you got mimicking? When were you last telling yourself how beautiful you are? Watch your bare breasts ever and tell yourself how beautiful you are? Remember: sex is one of the best slimming and cutting exercises. If you are fortunate enough to live with a partner, try to spice up your sex life. Many publications are available; just check what works for you. There's no cause to worry if you're alone. Sexual activity with your own self can be a fun and gentle workout, anytime and anywhere. Be your own best friend and lover—know what's going on, you know best.

3. Avoid sugar and empty carbohydrates: Sugar, white meal, rice, and other natural fiber free cereals will directly enter your blood from your stomach. They raise blood sugar levels and boost your energy until the sugar is consumed. Then you need some more sugar to boost you. A diet rich in sugar and empty carbohydrates keeps you eating all day, without feeling really satisfied and complete. The occasional ice cream, cookie, or pie, of course, is a pleasure to enjoy–but not a normal part of a healthy diet.

4. Eat a lot of food and drink plenty of water: this holds the metabolism together with exercise. You will never complain of constipation when you eat enough fiber and drink water at the same time. Healthy bowel movements are important to feel good. If your food stays in your body for too much time, waste accumulates. Don't forget to drink fiber water: fiber without moisture helps to coagulate the digestive system.

5. Take lactobacillus: the bacteria in your intestines help to break the food and feed your body so that it doesn't need to build up fat. You rarely complain about

bloating or excessive gas when you take lactobacillus each day in one form or another. Lactobacillus is available today in many ways, and she finds all sorts of problems extremely helpful. Take capsules if you don't like eating curd or other milk products.

6. Evite big meals: It's, of course, good to have a five- or six-course meal at times when you celebrate or just feel like it. Without indulgences, what would life be? However, it is better to keep your food smaller every day and eat more often. Disseminate your daily calorie intake and don't eat too late.

7. Avoid hunger pangs: don't wait until you're starving, keep eating. When your stomach grumbles and something you really need to eat, you tend to eat too fast. Our brain takes about 20 minutes to record that we have filled our stomachs so that it helps to eat slowly and to chew carefully.

8. Satisfy the cravings: try to satisfy this impulse when something makes the mouth water. Your body tells you what it has to do. Cravings are one of the manifestations of our bodies. As already stated: When

you feel like eating strawberries (or hot dogs or chocolate bars), do what you want.

9. Vitamins and minerals: Make sure you get enough vitamins and minerals to your doctor's advice by taking supplements.

10. Ultimately, the obvious thing: don't drink too much alcohol; eat enough fruit and vegetables and sleep enough. When you can't sleep well, feel tired or discontented, depression and/or hormone imbalance may be felt. Go to your doctor and get assistance.

Ease Into Your Diet For Stress Free Weight Loss Success

Depending on your height and how much body fat you have, in the first 3-4 weeks of any correctly structured nutrition program, you should expect to lose 6-20 pounds of body weight. In addition, a reasonable objective is to try and lose 2 pounds/week for the rest of the time. It means a realistic weight loss goal for 3-4 months is about 30-40 pounds. More than that is uncommon and possibly dangerous in this time frame and should only be done under close medical supervision if you have one hundred lbs. This can not normally be achieved in, for example, a 12-16 week program to lose; you will need more than one nutrition program to achieve this objective. If you need more than one diet, don't expect to do one after another because the returns are may. It's advisable to take a brief 1-2 week break between classes, but if you're going to lose more than 10-15 pounds, you can expect to suffer from a diet for months. It will be imperative to keep yourself as mentally fresh as possible during your journey.

Given the length of time required to produce fat loss results on a diet, it is intelligent to make it easier and to apply measures throughout that will prevent your burning. Even if you are very excited to start your new diet, do not immerse yourself in the cold turkey approach and try to follow your plans to the' T' from the outset. If you have 12 difficult weeks ahead, starting too tightly too quickly begins to wane far before the end of hunger and mental stress. If you are very long overweight or lose over 30 pounds of corporal fat, cold turkey can even be risky. If you have not done so (or have not done so in a very long time), eating completely clean and/or exercising will release toxins contained in the body's fat. You can get sick and even hurt if you do it too fast. Dietarians who have excessive body fat should make it easier for them to stop damaging their bodies with the rapid toxin dumping that can take place from beginning a too strict diet. An example is when an obese person starts a drastic 85 percent raw diet, changing dramatically from highly processed food to almost nothing but raw vegetables. Few can do it without getting ill. This is not advisable as a result can be very dangerous.

They say that for 21 days, you must do the same before it becomes a custom. Once you have hit the three-week mark on your diet, several techniques can make it much easier to keep up the race on the long distance. The trick is to ease your eating habits so that it is not difficult for you to get sick or mentally break down before reaching the 21-day habit area. The best way to do this is to take the first ten days, or even 2-3 weeks, and obey it, gradually getting tougher until you do everything in the book soon. This can be done in many ways. One option is to have a strict diet for several days, followed by a day or two off of the diet.

Start the first week with Monday, Wednesday, and Friday diets and take off for the rest of the days. The second week of diets is primarily planned for Monday and Tuesday, off Wednesday, Thursday, Friday, and Saturday, off Sunday. Three-week diet throughout the week and take a half-day off the diet as a reward on Saturday. The fourth week should be a strict diet for the rest of the program.

Another way to make a long weight loss program easier is the removal method. This is likely the most common and probably the safest way to start a diet, especially if you lose large amounts of weight. Instead of alternating strict days with days off in the first 2-3 weeks, take this time to remove poor food while adding good food. For example, eat all the processed sugars and bread for the first week instead of a strict diet with controlled servings; replace with only clean, complex starches, such as brown rice, yams / sweet potatoes, oats, and legumes. Replace all your liquids and increase your drinking water to at least 64 ounces/day, but almost a gallon/day if you are sweating hard enough. If you eat out, for week one, you will choose plain chicken breasts, lean steaks, plain potatoes, and salads. Week two, every meal is replaced by only prepared home-cooked meals for every meal containing the right quantity of protein but not limited in calories. Week 3 starts limited calorie meals and strict diets until the program's end.

In addition to easing your diet, it is also a good idea to make your workout easier. In order to effectively burn body fat, jumping into the head can also produce negative effects. Juggling strength and cardiovascular work is like taking a second job unexpectedly, which can easily work you, particularly when you're new to the fitness center. Just like your nutrition program, do your exercise for the first 1-2 weeks. If you're not used to strength training, start with a small volume for the first few sessions very moderately. If you don't do this, it will be difficult to avoid muscular soreness, overwhelming, discouraging, and closely monitoring or training. Go for a number of cardio hours/week and build it up over time. For starters, weeks one do 3 30 minute cardio sessions. Week two, do two 40 minute one 30 minute sessions and continue building up to 5-6 hours per week (or whatever your effective work volume maybe) in a number of sessions and duration.

Another reason why your nutrition program involves cold turkey is wrong is because of the unnecessary mental stress it adds. Most weight loss plans are successful because they are consistent with your scheme over a period of time. Feeling utterly unforgiving for 12 tough weeks allows any mental breakdown without at least some form of temporary relief. It takes a couple of weeks to ease the mental stress of diet for longer periods. Spending time on your diet also helps greatly with this type of stress. Follow your diet as strictly as possible throughout the week for the best results, but reward yourself with a cheat meal on the weekend. This allows you to work for, look forward to and satisfy your appetite. It also rests your mind and renews your eagerness to start fresh next week. Instead of always trying to see the light at the end of the tunnel, have a meal at a time and one day at a time. Focusing on the process instead of just on the product will keep your mind focused on a series of numerous small victories. Soon you will have spent enough time developing habits and seeing results.

Weight Loss - Tracking the Elusive Calorie

Do you know what you eat? What do you eat?

To show how easily we "forget" what we have eaten, try writing a log of what you ate from memory yesterday. You can remember the main meals, but it will probably be more difficult to remember the little bits here and there. You might even think you haven't had anything except the food, but most people do it, and yes, chewing gum counts, and you do whatever you put into your mouth. List the basic foods, meals, and so on as best you can remember. Then put it aside and write down what you actually eat when you eat it as soon as possible.

When you eat, don't write your log either. That's not you, and it's a prescribed diet that dictates. If you follow a certain plan, that's all right, but wait until you eat it to write it down. If you remember what you ate today, write that down too, including that tiny snack of cake as you passed and that tiny pick of the peanut dish. You must list everything you eat or drink, including simple water.

Such extra tastes and treats can easily add up to 250 calories or more each day. Especially if you taste while cooking. Here's a diet tip: stop liquidating your spoon! If you quit these little tastes while cooking, you can save this winter by adding a few pounds.

I know it sounds impossible, but just stops laughing the beaters, scratching the last bits, and popping bits in your mouth to "see if they're gone." Please wait for it, then go ahead and eat some, just note that those tastes add up and they won't be worth bringing about five extra pounds. Place mixing spoons and beaters underwater immediately, if necessary, or offer the children as a treat.

The point of a food journal is to capture the regular patterns of eating, and then choose one thing to change. It is easier to change one little habit at a time. No, not every single thing can cause great weight loss, but it adds up.

Now resolve to drop the habit of liking or tasting the spoon while you are cooking. I can hear you wailing that if it tastes right, you will not know. All right, so you need a little teensy taste, but not hundreds, get it? A small bit on a spoon or fork tip is not the same as many large bites during cooking. Tasting doesn't eat. The rest of the content of the bowl you used to make pudding is also not the same as the taste. This is a service. This is a service. It's better to break the habit. Yeah, when you were a kid, it's a holdover. It was a joy to lick the spoon, but you're no longer a kid? Let your children have their turn, but allow yourself this habit.

Remember, these small changes create real results. It is a trick of those who remain slender naturally. You can also choose one thing completely to change, discard or cut back, when you discover your general eating habits. Sometimes it's best to take it slowly as if you were weaning from whole milk to skim. Try 4% first, and if that seems all right, turn to 2% again. You will eventually drink skim milk and think it's okay, actually once you become used to it, you will think like pure cream of whole milk tastes.

Of course, whole milk tastes better than skim, so you taste thousands more than one other food, but you have to choose what you eat regularly. Would you like to eat a lot of calories and fat in your food, or would you prefer to eat something bigger than meat?

Many Would Starve if McDonald's went away from the business. What if there was a global energy shortage, and there were no quick food restaurants anymore? Would you curl in a ball and not know what else to eat or just learn what else to eat?? I will risk you adapting to the circumstances. Take a look at the "Confidential Restaurant" to see how many calories a regular meal in a restaurant has to offer. When you see that you eat three times as many calories as you can, it's a lot easier to eat every night or three times a week, twice or once, until one day you find that you eat only for special occasions.

I hardly eat anything! I hardly eat anything! How can I not lose weight?

I hear from many people who tell them that they can't understand why they can't lose weight but eat out in restaurants or have easy food two or more times a day. Simply don't you realize that you probably eat well over 2000 calories a day, and if you're not really active, you can add a few extra pounds. It's not nice to see how many calories you need to lose weight and then surpass the amount because you don't pay attention to it.

It takes some effort to monitor what you eat, but it's a great way to discover what's happening about your habits and triggers.

You can find that you hit the candy dish six times a day or chew a whole bunch of gum every day. You could use only one or two additional soft drinks or coffee drinks to consume hundreds of calories every day. Many coffee beverages actually contain over 500 calories each. Usually, that's more than you would eat for your whole breakfast.

Begin with just a small blank notebook. If you like the process, you might want to look into a software program, but the sooner you begin yourself, the sooner you'll succeed in losing weight.

CHAPTER SIX:
Lifestyle Changes Needed For Effective Weight Loss

Most people were once looking for that perfect diet to achieve successful weight loss. The triste truth is that most dietitians fail. This was because the decreased calorie diet lasting months or weeks is often accompanied by a return to your old bad habits. You have to make permanent lifestyle changes to keep the weight off. A few proven strategies:

Achieve effective Weight Loss By Making Daily Workouts a Habit

In just three weeks ' time, you can develop a habit. Consistency is the key. Prepare your workout every day at the same time. When you miss a day or two, stick to the routine rather than give up.

You can't lose weight effectively without resistance training in your workouts. This gives your body lean, toned muscles and increases your metabolism, too. You can lose more weight in the long run and keep it off. Strong muscles also allow for more efficient movement and injury prevention. Cardio should also be included in your workouts. Cardio training strengthens the heart and blood vessels, increasing your stamina.

During your workouts, remember to rest between exercises for no more than 30 seconds. This will dramatically lead to a larger calory burn than to remain between exercises for more than 30 seconds.

To achieve an effective weight loss, cultivate a physically active lifestyle instead of driving. Swap the driveway for parking and walking. Choose and walk away from your destination and parking spaces. Swap sedentary hobbies like active gaming, such as skateboarding or gardening. You will burn more calories, keep healthy, and significantly improve your chances of successful weight loss through more physical activity in your everyday life.

Get successful weight loss by cooking more at home

28% of Americans say they don't know how to cook. If you are eating and eating a diet of convenience, it is far harder to eat a wide range of healthy foods. Learn how to cook and buy fresh food to control your diet regularly.

Eating late-night snacks

Does not lead to significant weight loss. At least three hours before bedtime, you should finish your last meal. Throughout sleep, your metabolism decreases, and your body changes from fat burning to fat storage, which can result in weight gain and sleep cycle variability. Moreover, you might need to get up and urinate more. If you must eat late, eat food that is low in calories and high in whole grains.

Eat A Healthy Breakfast

One of the biggest factors to achieve an effective weight loss is breakfast daily. Breakfast is the biggest meal of the day. Breakfast gives you the fuel you need to boost your day. In a recent study, people who had breakfast lost an average of 18 pounds over three months for the biggest meal of the day. Other people who participated in the study ate the exact number of calories per day, but they ate most calories during dinner.

Drink Plenty Of Water

Why does it take enough water every day to lose weight effectively? Simply put, water decreases the hunger and increases the capacity of the body to burn stored fat. Research has shown that an inadequate intake of water causes fat deposits to increase across the body, while adequate amounts of water can reduce fat deposits.

This happens because the kidneys can't function properly when you don't drink enough water. The liver must, therefore, step up and perform some of the functions of the kidneys. One of the major functions of the liver is to separate stored fat chemically into energy for the body to use. However, when the liver has to perform certain kidney functions, it can not metabolize as much fat. Therefore, less fat is consumed, and more weight is added. It is recommended to drink 8 to 12 glasses of water per day on average. If you are a very active person, increasing this number.

Learn to love healthy foods

A whole diet tastes strange to you at first when you are used to eating high fat salty and processed foods. Learn a range of healthy ways of preparing fresh foods. Toss it in olive oil before roasting in melted cheese or butter instead of drowning broccoli. Instead of salt, choose lemon juice, hot sauce, and spices to add a flavor. Then, leave the soda out. Just by eliminating heavily sweetened drinks from your diet, you can change your preferences to choose healthy and natural foods. You should eat every three to four hours throughout the day-3 basic meals and two or more healthy snacks (fruit, nuts, dark chocolate, popcorn, peanut butter, and crackers, etc.). This will keep your metabolism up, lead to more calories being consumed, help to control your appetite, and make weight loss more effective.

Schedule A Rewards Day

Improve your drive to exercise regularly and eat healthy foods at least once a week. This award could be your favorite dessert, a weekend break, or a great play or musical experience.

Get Sleep Enough

The loss of sleep can lead to weight gain. Try to sleep for six to eight hours a night. The increase in weight is caused by a hormone, ghrelin, that increases as sleep loss occurs. Along with others, this hormone stimulates the brain to crave more fattening products such as French fries, chocolate chip cookies, and other sweets.

Eat Mindfully.

We can have hundreds of empty calories if we don't want snack chips or cookies because we're anxious, bored, or unhappy. Make the food the center of your attention when you sit down to eat. Taste every bite. Do not eat or work while watching TV. By eating carefully, you will find yourself more satisfied and eat less.

The most important point to remember when it comes to a successful weight loss is that long term success only comes when you decide to make lifestyle changes that enable you to make the best choices about good food and regular exercise. Basically, these decisions will decide the quality of your life.

Better Body Composition Or Simple Weight Loss?

A good friend of mine once said that it was easy to lose weight. Lock yourself for some days in a closet, and you're going to drop lots of weight. Quite far-fetched, but he was right with the idea of weight loss. People come to me usually to ask for a solution to weight loss, but what they want is a change in body composition. The difference between simple weight loss and change in body composition is a good idea. The ability to differentiate them ensures that you understand and choose the right course to achieve and maintain results. For many readers, this may seem like technical surveillance that will have no effect, but it is a very important distinction. Let's look at the fundamental definition of both here in fitness. Losing weight simply reduces any weight of the body. Body mass consists of fat mass (FM), and free fat mass (FFM). This includes a wide variety of connective tissues, bones, muscles, organs, and body fluids. Any day a person can temporarily gain and lose 3 pounds of weight without changing daily conduct. So we can already see how unstable the weight-loss idea can be.

A person can create or maintain a good composition of the body in the fitness industry by maintaining or gaining FFM when losing FM. One major difference in weight loss and changes in body composition is that a change in composition can or can not change a person's weight. Thus, someone could lose pounds of fat and not lose any weight on the scale. This is attributable to the respective FM-FFM ratio. A person can gain muscle and water while losing fat, without changing weight. A person can also lean while maintaining or even gaining weight. Once, because of the FFM to FM radio. Another way of looking at it is to spread fat mass across the body. It takes more room than the fat-free mass. Fat mass is lighter than muscle mass, too. Weight can then be lost, and muscles can be retained or added, which creates no change in body weight, but the body's size and shape change for the better.

Now that we have a handle of each let's see why you focus better on improving the makeup of the body than simply losing weight. The so-called doctor-supported weight loss clinics and promoted fitness franchises appear everywhere in daring posters displaying a skinny person holding giant pants with the slogan "lose

50 lb in four weeks." It's probable and quite serious. The unfortunate part is weight loss simply means losing different body masses (not just fat) in order to achieve more weight. Therefore, without regard to better body shape, the ability to sustain weight loss is impossible. Many who concentrate on weight loss, regardless of the healthy body's makeup, end up with the effects of decreased metabolism, lowered sex drive, increased fat ratios, and the "skinny-fat structure."

As extreme weight loss tactics are unstable, the dreaded "snap back" reaction will be very likely to occur after the diet is complete. Many times, if not more, a person gains the weight back. The human body's homeostasis will not change unless it is necessary to survive. If you are an athlete or have some other active and challenging lifestyle, your body may not have to change a lot to survive. Let's tell you a clear example by saying that someone loses weight with a diet endorsed by an extreme doctor and the typical aerobics classes. She quickly loses weight. The skin shrinks a little, she feels more miserable and hasn't kept much muscle, so she's slender and fat. Obviously, by the party a few days, she enjoys her new fat body and soon starts binge snacking. One month later, our not but obese is fat. She returns very soon to receive additional supplements and injections from her extreme weight loss clinicians, and after a few weeks, she leaves the program and again begins to bing. When this instance decided to lose weight through aerobic activities such as aerobic classes, she found, together with extreme diets, that the body still does not require enough to prevent fuel cannibalization and fat loss of the muscle. Although the example is fictional, I have always seen it. The morality of the story, an easy and very unstable loss of weight, can happen quickly, but it simply doesn't consider the side effects of a bad mood, poor joint and bone health, reduced metabolism, lower sex drive, and fat stockpiling. As you can see, weight loss is pretty worthless without respect for body composition.

Conversely, it is a great idea to change the makeup of the body for the better. Changing the composition of the body would mean supporting as much FFM as possible and would also increase it for many. The FFM encourages optimum metabolism and can sustain an active level. Nevertheless, this sort of shift can not always be achieved by just looking every day in the mirror. It is, therefore, possible to use various measuring instruments to collect sound information. As bodybuilder trainer Christian Thibadeau once pointed out, there are certain points where there is no change in the mirror while losing fat. In general, this area ranges between 18-15% of male body fat and 25-19% female. The data you obtain on your body speaks for itself at this level.

Dieting is nothing In Losing Weight

So many people want to know how to lose weight, but why is it so hard to continue to eat? Everybody seems to know that nutritional weight loss is almost impossible to achieve (and still more difficult to maintain), but millions of people still do not spend billions of pounds a year in the expectation that the Holy Grail-a diet that actually works for the normal people-is found. There needs to be a better way...

First, why are diets failing? The main reason is that you focus on one thing you can't have' going on a diet.' When you were told as a child you couldn't have any sweets, what was the one thing you wanted? It is human nature to want the things we most often think about. So if you're' on a diet' that means you can't have any pasta, you're just thinking of pasta all over the planet. Your willpower will fail sooner or later, and you will break only once. Then again and again... And again...

Another diététic question is that the dietitian finds the diet a panacea. "I'm on a diet, so I don't have to do anything else in order to lose weight." Well, sorry, that's not true. In reality, a diet can, in one way, make things worse. Most dietitians note a loss of energy and excitement. The effect is that they are less physically active than before. Thus even if you can consume fewer calories by being "good" and sticking to your diet, you also use fewer calories and, therefore, either don't lose weight or not as much as you should.

So how do you manage to make a real difference? I would love to say that you can buy a pill that's going to drop the pounds. Or you can learn a special technique to lose weight from the convenience of your own couch. But I can't, sadly. I know you want to lose weight because, as you have spent a fortune on diets, you even have to read this segment down, and still don't know if it could be beneficial. The fact is that you have to do some work. It won't be difficult, but it will take a little effort.

The most important thing to know is that if you use more calories than you use at the simplest level, you get more weight, and you lose weight when using more calories than you consume. You can examine this to the millionth degree and worry that' fat calories' have more effect than' carbohydrate calories,' or whether the glycaemic food index affects the digestion rate, which is... And so on. And so on. However, you can not escape the fact that eating more calories than you are using will make your weight.

We already know that most people don't try to cut their calorie intake easily. The only way is to try using more calories. If you think about going to the fitness center and how to work hard and drag, it will live up to your expectations. If you think of the sexy, slender, and slimming, you work towards, and on the other hand, you will have a very good image in your mind to help remove your mind from the exercise. I'm not in favor of joining a gym. Of course not, but we'll come later on!

Getting physically active works in several ways: you use more calories by being more active, so you can create a calorie deficit that is what you need to lose weight.

Also, since you're going to be on your feet more and do more things, your mind and body won't have enough time to think about the food you've missed. So, of course, you tend to snack less, and you don't even notice it.

When you increase your activity level, your body begins to adapt. If you want to walk more, your leg muscles must be bigger than if you're sitting down all your life. So the exercise begins to increase the muscle you have. Muscle takes more energy to maintain than fat, making your metabolism grow with more muscle. You now use more calories than you did when you had a higher fat ratio, even while sitting down!

I notice that being more healthy makes me want less to feed. Perhaps it's because of the stress in your stomach muscles. I really don't know. I know I tend to eat smaller portions. I know. I still eat the same stuff, but I don't feel like that much. So the consumption of calories, therefore decreases.

There are good reasons, psychologically and physically, why more exercise is more likely to work than just a diet. There are also other good reasons. Studies show that starting to exercise for 30 minutes a day, five days a week is the best thing you can do for your health. The advantages are so numerous that they need a product of their own but begin by reducing the risk of heart disease and diabetes, and continue to benefit a large number of other health benefits that you can not get by changing the food that you eat.

So how can you begin? The easiest way is to walk. Go five days a week for a 30-minute walk. If you can't do it, continue with what you can do. Make sure you do it at least five days a week. The human body is a wonderful thing and adapts to its surroundings. So even if you don't have the time to start 30 minutes a day, your body can adjust periodically so that you can gradually increase the time, and then finally reach this target.

Then every time you start to walk faster until you walk briskly. Fast enough to get your pulse rate up, warm your body, and breathe deeper. Generally, you'll feel fitter at this point and almost definitely lose some weight. The fact that you feel so much more comfortable will motivate you to keep going and develop more. Since you know then how to lose weight and how to get fitter, the sky is the limit. Would you like to run a marathon? Why not! Why not!

If Diets and Weight Loss Programs Leave You Cold - Start Your Own!

A DIET NOT IS A PERMANENT LOSS SOLUTION

Dieting, which removes some things from your normal food list, which is only certain foods you eat or eat, does not function as a permanent weight loss solution. This could be explained in a book itself, but in short, you get tired, it's difficult for you to remain on a diet because diet induces body changes which encourages weight gain, you are losing energy, it's simply not enjoyable, etc. Choose any diet you want. Pick any diet. Were you prepared to eat like this for the rest of your life? Perhaps not. A change in lifestyle and behavior is the only real solution to a lifetime problem.

DIETS ARE MISUNDERSTOOD AND MISHANDLED.

The classic example here is the Atkins diet! Tell almost anyone you're aware of Atkins ' diet, and they'll tell them it's a diet that allows us to eat plenty, such as steaks, burgers, and you know, nice, without thinking about the nasty old vegetables and carbohydrates. You will know from a few pages in the Atkins diet plan that eating like this should only take about the first two weeks in order to push the body in proper mode for the next three stages.

Ironically, Atkins Diet and almost every other weight loss plan, fitness coach, diet pill, diet drink, you name it, incorporates exercise as a key to its success.

You HAVE TO EXERCICE TO WEIGHT LOSS

Many people might actually lose the majority of our weight by getting in and staying with the right exercise program! This is half the problem. Half the problem.

Our bodies are designed to do Things by Mother Nature! Remote clicking doesn't count.

The basic rule of weight loss and weight gain is that you get weight if you eat more calories than you burn. You lose weight because you eat more calories than you burn. That easy. That simple.

It really seems easy for most people. When you eat less, you are going to lose weight!

TO SUBSTITUTE OF GOOD NUTRITION

As mentioned above, simply cutting food from your diet is not the solution. The answer, however, is easy-just eat sensibly. Nobody ever said you couldn't eat chocolate cake, you just shouldn't eat 2 to 3 pieces a day, and it should be a small slice you DO consume. We all have a vague idea at least of what food we SHOULD consume and a good idea of what not to eat or at least to eat a lot. It's an active process. Many people ride to the window and say, "Bring me your 99-cent greaseburger and a cup of water with sugar." When you ask, "supersize it," you accept. Even the good restaurants serve a lot more food than they are healthy to eat, but most people eat it anyway because they don't know what to do because it tastes so well or because they have been taught to clean their dishes.

You see lots of diet and weight loss items claiming to have found THE SOLUTION to your weight loss problem. Thanks to one single thing, hardly anyone is overfat (Arnold Schwarzenegger is "overweight"). Most of the time, it will occur because of a combination of factors. While nutrition and exercise are two important MOST absolute factors, simply changing one without the other does not work, and both are implemented. Slight things like an electric exercise belt, a grapefruit pill, or a Tahiti secret drink that support your weight loss program, but don't expect to see a lot about the results if you aren't already doing the two most important things. There is good scientific evidence that things like cortisol and caffeine, for example, can affect weight gain and weight loss, but if you were to try to control weight for a lifetime by regulated those factors, you would be able to find out that these items have a significant impact on the label, which says something like... when they are used with a proper diet and a regular exercise. If you are, however, to start eating sensibly and exercising, taking cortisol blockers or cutting caffeine out of your diet, then MIGHT contributes a couple of pounds of extra weight loss, but you are likely to lose weight if your weight loss program continues.

YOUR WEIGHT LOSS PROGRAM THAT'S THE GOAL You are not your parent, sister, or mother regardless of how closely you genetically associate with them. Perhaps it isn't what fits for one of them. While there is scientific evidence to support the equations described above, each person will react in his or her own way. You must practice, but perhaps not as much as your friend. You will consume less ice cream, but you may not be able to eat as much as your friend does. Through constructing it around you, you will make every weight loss program work for you. Make sure you do enough of the exercises you like to do. What's enough? What's enough? Well, you're going to have to experiment and see. Eat the foods you like, just eat them in sensible amounts and eat mainly foods with a lot of real nutrition. What foods? What foods? Again, probably by trial and error, you have to find a way, although there are plenty of excellent books to guide you.

When it comes to goals, the goal is to be healthy and happy. You want to weigh a certain weight because someone else bears the weight is meaningless. You shouldn't even try to weigh what you weighed in high school because that was a different person physically speaking. He or she had a different appetite, a different lifestyle, and different tastes. Concentrate on getting your workout and eating well and let your body realize how much it wants more weight.

Trying to customize a weight loss program for the performance of someone else just calls for issues in terms of weight loss. You can run faster than you can. You can have a metabolic rate higher than you. They may have a different structure of the bone. You may have fewer obstacles than you do. Faced with this, someone such as Brad Pitt and Angelina Jolie can have the best equipment, the finest personal trainer, and can sculpt a beautiful body. Therefore, they have the opportunity to realize that their multimillion-dollar salaries rely on maintaining their genetic make-up. You and I have an old set of barbells, a broken pavement, shoes falling down, paycheck alive, children's home in two hours. You and I will not look like Brad, Angelina, or Arnold. Just do your best with what you have, and you won't regret the result, trust me.

CHAPTER SEVEN:
Weight Loss And Metabolism

From time to time, there are things you hear. They seem common words or sentences, you tie them to a certain topic, and you even think you understand what it means. Sometimes, however, you don't know the meaning of the word and how it really relates to the subject with which you have come.

One of these words is "metabolism." In the supermarket check-out line, magazines have titles like "This food can improve your metabolism." "Your metabolism has slowed down in the last few years," your physician says. You also hear a new "ultra metabolism" weight-loss craze.

From those and a few hundred other situations, you found out that metabolism has something to do with weight loss and weight gain, but do you really know what the relationship is? These are three questions that we will try to answer quickly, but with enough detail to improve the weight loss program.

WHAT IS METABOLISM?

Metabolism can be described as a word or process in two simple statements. First, it's your body's chemical process for sustaining life, giving energy and forming vital substances such as blood, bone, muscle, fat, etc. Secondly, specific substances of its processing, such as fat iodine, metabolism, and many more. While these two apply to what we speak about, the first statement is currently relevant for you.

YOUR METABOLISM IS HOW YOUR BODY

absorbs energy from food and constructs and replaces tissue and organs, and how it functions effectively. The last section on performance is a key element of weight loss and weight gain.

What is the METABOLISM
Related to what we are... and we are gaining?

Your metabolism worked in different ways at different times in your life. A lot of you remember the days when you could eat something you wanted and never get a pound. A great pizza, three sugar sodas, and some cinnamon sticks, no change at all!

Your metabolism is in the higher gears in the younger years of your life, probably the highest gears ever. Weight gain and weight loss are not really problems for most of you in these years. Nevertheless, some people have slower metabolic rates and genetic factors or health conditions, which cause them to gain weight more than others in their age group. Either the community you are within will increase the speed and efficiency with which your body turns food into energy and body "part and half" by increasing your metabolic rate, reviving your metabolism.

Sadly, your metabolism has slowed down as you aged for a long time. Part of this is just something that the body does with age; while partly age-related, it is the effect of changes that take place in your age way of life. Fortunately, both are reversible, mainly in the same process. More in the last section. The portion that slows down the body has to do with the "rest metabolism," and the other half... Ok, let's just call it "resting metabolism."

RESTING METABOLISM

The body still has some home-keeping tasks to do when you are doing something that doesn't seem to require energy. Your diaphragm expands and contracts, and your heart, for instance, pumps blood. Tissues are replaced, and waste is taken away. As you sit in a semi-vegetative state, your body is working hard.

This restful metabolic rate declines as you age. At least one estimate puts the reduction between childhood and retirement at about 10% and another 10% after that. The odds are that your body does not change into the energy it used to like pizza and soda and cinnamon sticks. Your internal maintenance is not as efficient as it used to be, so after the meal, there is usually some more "thing" left in the air when you were a teenager. This decrease happens to almost everyone, so if you have no weight problem at high school, you may see your body build up with fat as you grow old. In your younger years, if you DID have a weight problem, it will probably only get worse.

UNDERESTABLISHING YOUR METABOLISM AS PART OF YOUR LOSS PROGRAM

Having learned about the metabolism of rest and rusting could tend to eat less. To tell the truth, knocking a few calories out of the diet might be enough for a quick, short-term weight loss. Such missing pounds must eventually come home, though, and possibly bring some mates with them and diets have additional problems not discussed here. One of the things that you need to know is that if your diet makes your caloric intake below a certain point for a certain time, your body adapts its metabolic rate to a new, permanent, lower level and not only keeps your weight below the calories but can also start to increase the weight again. If you go off that calorie-limited diet, your body will continue to chug with fewer calories, and your weight will return up, perhaps even higher than it used to be. Since your metabolism is now lower, the next time you lose weight will be even more difficult.

TIP: Although a diet may not respond, you're probably eating items you could do without or in excess of what you need if you're a normal 21st-century person. For example, sugar. Just look at that tub of ice cream. The last I saw was 16 servings. There were 16 servings. A couple of years ago, one of those boxes lasted four times for me. Take a look around, and you can make a few improvements.

EXERCISE BURNS CALORIES You hardly change the resting rate of your remote control for changing TV channels. You have just.... oh my God as you get up and walk across your room to change the channel and go back to your chair.trained.... trained. It's not just that, you have burnt a few more calories just by getting you... I was... out of the chair, sorry. Go riding, fishing, cooking, hiking, talking to the house. If public practice embarrasses you, blame the dog! "Yes, the vet said he needed to get more out of it. HE's putting a couple of pounds on it." Is nobody going to think you walk... right? Whatever it is, do it every day, or at least many times a week, and some extra calories and pounds of fat you'll burn off.

YOUR RESTING METABOLIC RATE IS RAISED BY EXERCISE

Most fitness exercises, typically of anaerobic type, take place in the course of time. The tendency to move the body to a higher rate of metabolic. You can lose some extra calories while walking if you go out for a long walk today. Take this long walk every day for several weeks, and your restful metabolic rate will actually rise, and if you are in front of the television, you will burn more calories. Not only will your metabolic rates be higher for a while after you complete the workout, but you will also continue to consume excess calories for a short period of time instead of just consuming excess calories during the exercise.

Other sports, such as resistance, create lean muscle mass. Muscle tissue burns more calories than other tissue types, like fat tissue, and creating magic muscle mass will not just burn calories during exercise, but the magical muscle mass incorporated into your body will keep burning calories, increasing your remaining metabolic rate.

TIP: Excess calories will be burnt daily, and your metabolism will increase. Changing some of your eating habits, such as removing unnecessary fats and carbs (yes, some fats are needed) and looking at portion sizes, will reduce your body's excess calories.

This double-barred strategy gives you the most powerful lifelong experience of weight loss.

Weight Loss and Your Health

Look no more for a complete and accurate guideline for weight reduction. This chapter will guide you to the most intelligent and successful behavior for a safer and sexier body. For comparison with other recommendations concentrating only on one part of the diet, this section will include all you need to know about reducing weight.

You have to understand how the body process works before following a diet or exercise. The body is capable of performing its daily function at a calorie maintenance level. The right amount of calories helps you to walk and retain your inner body functions. Calories are the source of power for the body. You will feel sick without the right amount of calories.

Our drinking and eating habits are the calories we need. The weight does not increase or decrease whether we consume the same amount of calories to suit our daily needs. Demonstrate this: if you eat 3,000 calories a day and you consume the same amount every day, you won't increase your weight when we consume more than our calorie maintenance level, weight increases. The opposite happens when we use the daily maintenance level. We can also reduce calories by eating less of our daily maintenance. A person with a quantity of 3000 calories should, therefore, consume 2500 calories to reduce weight.

I'm sure you'd like to understand your calorie maintenance degree at this moment. Your maintenance degree is determined by the Harris-Benedict Equation's Basal Metabolic Rate (BMR). The BMR of the body is the number of calories that you need to eat in order to continue your daily tasks. How much activity you do is taken into account when calories are calculated that you must burn every day. You can search online for daily calorie calculators to understand what your body needs.

Now that you understand the principle behind weight reduction, it is time to know the basic ways of losing weight. These three main ways are all you need. The first thing is to do it. You can burn more calories by exercising. If you commit to maintaining your daily calories, you will end up losing the same amount. Therefore, no weight change occurs. But if you want to reduce weight, you will have to exercise that removes more of the maintenance level of your calories. In the previous example, you will have to reduce weight loss by 500 additional calories.

Including workout, you must also eat less of your daily maintenance. Those with 3000 maintenance will have to sacrifice five hundred calories and eat only five hundred. There is a caloric shortage when you give your body fewer calories for maintenance. The body's steady weight loss would result in more food shortages.

The safest and most recommended weight loss method calls for both diet and workout. Eating fewer calories and burning more calories gives your body the stability of what your activities have gained and lost. It was consistently confirmed that a healthy diet and workouts would result in faster and longer-lasting weight loss.

The use of both methods is also the right way and does not interfere with your daily responsibilities.

Before you enter a workout or diet, you first need to analyze the maintenance level of your body. The study will change the form to a better routine. Start by regularly eating your calorie maintenance every day. Sustain food consumption for 2 to 3 weeks. It doesn't have to be the same amount of calories as long as it's close. To ensure that you are eating a suitable amount, weigh yourself at the start of the day once a week (before you eat and on an empty stomach).

If you have a stable weight for two to three weeks, you can eat the calories you need at the maintenance level. You must eat 500 less of your daily maintenance level per day to reduce your weight. If your maintenance level is 2500, only 2000 calories per day will need to start to be consumed.

Those who could not sustain their rate of calorie consumption can still continue a healthy weight loss program. All you have to do is take 500 less maintenance and adjust your body to the smaller quantity of calories. If you have succeeded in eating the lower maintenance level, you must again consume less than 500 of the initial amount.

It is crucial that you don't lose weight too quickly. Reducing weight at a dangerous pace can jeopardize your safety. If you get three or more pounds lossed regularly each week for a few weeks in a row, you will need to make some adjustments. The modification contains between 250 and 300 calories for your everyday use. After that, you have to check the new quantity for your weight. You shouldn't only eat a smaller amount, remember. You must practice reducing enough calories to reduce your weight.

The weight reduction level recommended is roughly 1 to 2 pounds per week. Remember, weight reduction will not benefit your body very quickly. You must maintain a loss pace that keeps you fit. Your wellbeing is far more critical than it looks good. Our mechanics can not recover from a very rapid weight loss. Ultimately, it just changes to stay alive if you speed up the procedure. Instead, body fat is preserved so that it can catch up. Then, you just have to stick to shed 1 to

2 pounds a week. If you can do that for one year, you can eventually lose between fifty and 100 pounds!

As we have covered the equations already, it's time to get to the specifics. What kind of meals do you eat? What do you have to avoid at all costs?

Let's begin with the positive side. There is a lot of delicious food that allows you to maintain and lose weight. Don't fall into fading diets that say that low carbs or no fats can give you the best results. Such diets are just for the sake of your desperation. All foods are required for a balanced physical. You only need to align them accordingly. The best experts to talk to our physicians and nutritionists about food choices. They give your money value and only look for your health.

A good diet requires the right amount of fats, carbohydrates, and proteins. An average healthy adult needs 30% of its calorie intake from fat. Therefore, 400 to 600 calories will be fat if you eat 2000 calories daily. Because nine calories are contained in 1 g of fat, the average person will eat 44 to 66 g per day.

Nuts, seeds, olive and canola oil, avocados, fish, fish oil, and flax-oil formulas are the best sources of fat. Weight reducers should be mindful that fat does not really make you "fat" if it is extracted from healthy foods. Fat won't get in the way of your loss of weight. It will only improve your health and endurance. You won't have to worry as long as you get your fat from the above sources.

Carbohydrates are another infamous food type for faded dieters. It is recommended that 50% of your calorie intake is filled with carbs. The conversion you have to note is: four calories are one gram of carbohydrates. Therefore, someone who eats 2000 calories per day will eat a thousand carbohydrates. So you have 250 grams of carbohydrates to eat a day. Healthy carbs include bananas, sweet potatoes, bohemian beans, tomatoes, oatmeal, and brown rice. In other words, eat complex carbohydrates rather than simple carbohydrates. Simple carbohydrates consist of sucrose foods such as white rice, white bread, soda, and other processed food.

The minimum daily level recommended for protein is 0.8 grams per kg of your body weight. Divide the weight by 2.2 and subtract by 0.8 to measure this. Since this is the minimum, people taking part in the training will consume more than the measured quantity. To ensure your safety, you can eat a little more. Protein choices include turkey, chicken, fish, maggot meat, white eggs, nuts, and beans.

Let's go to the food you need to avoid. Obviously, most of these foods are very bad for your well-being. Soft drinks, fast food, candy, cookies, crackers, cakes, baked goods, and chips are all basics not to eat. Besides these, don't eat trans and saturated fat foods. Stay away from foods containing increased levels of sodium and sugar. These meals typically contain your additional calories. In addition to the additional pounds, you will move to an unhealthy lifestyle.

Now that we talked about the diet, it's time to talk about exercise. The best way to burn calories is to work out. In addition to weight loss, it increases your strength, flexibility, and endurance. It will also help you to avoid heart disease and bone loss in the long term.

Two types of exercise are available: aerobic and anaerobic. Aerobic exercise is better known as aerobic workouts. Cardiovascular training improves your cardiovascular endurance with minimum to average strength at a lasting pace. Cardio activities include walking, skating, jogging, swimming, cycling, and elliptical machinery. The most prescribed exercise in cardiology is one you like and want to take part in habitually. Those who like to walk should walk every day. Bikers can continue their hobbies while swimming is perfect for water enthusiasts. The suggested schedule is 30 minutes in terms of time. Those who can carry on the above will proceed. However, the average person is recommended for thirty minutes. Perform aerobic exercise for approximately three to six days a week.

Anaerobic training works on your strength and stamina. Typically these are weight training, calisthenic training (such as pushups), and resistance equipment. Anaerobic activities give you a tremendous amount of calories. Although it isn't as much as aerobic preparation, it increases the stamina for cardio exercises. It will also give your body a very positive look. The muscle gain would make you look more toned and attractive. The recommended speed is two to four times a week for anaerobic exercises.

There are also some diet legends that must be ignored by everyone. The first is the myth that eating fat and carbohydrates makes you fat. Did we not simply say that fat and carbs are important to the health of a person? You need these types of foods to sustain your calories. The next one is stupid and useless diets. Just eating a little celery or chicken soup will kill you. Just eating a small meal won't burn your fat. Your body simply responds to food shortages and retains your fat.

Another myth is that workouts on spot reduction allow you to lose all your fats. It is not the solution to concentrate on a single area. This is because exercise relies on your muscles. If the muscles are covered with fat, they may remain hidden. You must get the fat to expose the muscles.

The most noticeable errors are the products sold in newspapers. Depending on one drug, people do not lose their weight. The same goes for ab computers. These machines are just another spot reduction case.

Any other quick or easy way to reduce weight is just to get your money. You have to accept that loss of weight involves perseverance and a great deal of time.

You should use a gym membership if you would like to save cash for your weight loss. Gyms have aerobic and anaerobic training equipment. It's also a good motivator. You wouldn't want to spend your money and not use it. You are also inspired by men. Something else helps you reduce weight: a digital food scale, a bicycle, an elliptical machine, weights, tape measurement, and a bodyweight scale.

You need to eat smaller foods more, usually in terms of your diet. Eating one to three big meals a day is not recommended. Bring it down into five to six small meals instead. Each 2 to 3 hours, eat meals. Another way to improve your diet is to prepare your food. Plan it early in the week and cook it early. You are thus not packed with fatty foods sold in restaurants or fast food. You should also eat with water. Drink it while you eat the meal. The water will fill you up more quickly and prevent you from using additional calories. Don't eat very quickly. The body takes a while to realize that it gets full. Gradually grind food and don't eat in a hurry. When you eat too much, you can eat more than your body does.

If you're just starting a weight loss routine, it's a long-term activity. You will have to hold this weight by measuring your progress and making the necessary measurements. Unless you forget, you're going to get all this weight too quickly. To be healthy is a way of life, a true commitment to the needs of your body.

A Simple Diet And Exercise Plan To Lose One Pound A Week

If you are ready to lose weight, so that you look sexier and healthier, then the best advice anyone can give is to understand the simple ways to lose one pound a week.

Understanding how to lose one pound a week helps you build the basis for a more healthy loss of weight.

Everyone who wants to lose weight usually wants to lose it or lose more weight over a short period of time than practical.

Begin to learn how to lose one pound a week and use this as a basis for additional weight loss.

A weight loss goal can be reached through an online or offline journal or notebook.

You can monitor what you eat, the number of calories, the workout, and how you feel that day with this device.

An excellent option is to create a simple online blog for yourself and to share every day updates on how your diet and practice plans went throughout the day. An online blog also allows you to easily navigate blogs on diet, exercise, and weight loss. These forums are full of members who try to lose weight, maintain weight, or have lost weight successfully. They can be a helpful and motivational tool as you want to formulate fresh and varied food choices, ways to exercise, and motivation to stick to your schedule.

When you do nothing else to change your level of activity every day and reduce your calorie intake by 500 calories, you start to lose weight. Depending on the amount you consume at the moment every day, you can find that your caloric intake is too reduced to keep comfortable. The same happens if you increase your calorie intake by 250 calories per day and proceed with the same level of activity, but this will result in a loss of only about half a pound per week.

The next move is to adjust the activity level so that you continue to eat enough calories to lose one pound a week. If your calorie intake has reduced by 250 calories, you actually have to raise your activity levels to consume 250 calories a day if you want to lose 1 pound a week.

What is your activity to burn 250 calories?

The first step is to evaluate your current level of activity and to find ways to get more involved without interfering with your daily routine or causing more tension.

Anything that disrupts your day increases your spending time away from your family or reduces your enthusiasm for stuff, which will eventually increase your level of stress every day. This additional stress will increase your chances of not adhering to your weight loss plan, so make sure you fit your current routine and mindset with whatever you do to increase your activity. Going to the gym is an excellent option, but if it takes 1-2 hours a day, you have to do other daily tasks, and family time, it will not be long before you make excuses to stop doing so.

Walking is one of the easiest ways to increase your level of activity.

Walking about an hour a day gives around 200 calories an hour, depending on how quickly you go.

If your job requires you to sit most of the day, then start standing up and walking during breaks and lunch. Consider taking the stairs to work during your lunch, and when you go home. Park far from the main entrance of your office if you can still walk safely. A simple change in your level of activity will help to burn the calories you lose 1 pound a week.

The success and failure of most weight loss plans come from the failure to stick to your diet or motivation to exercise and to exercise to reach your weight loss goals.

If you want to excel in weight loss, then learning how we gain and lose weight will allow you to keep track of your weight loss plan. You can then use that information. You will be more inclined to stick to your diet and weight loss program rather than to quit frustration because you know that over time you'll start watching pounds fall. It increases your self-esteem and helps you to stick to the weight loss program.

You also have to find how to choose the right foods, how to prepare the right foods, how often to eat, why exercise is a must, how much exercise and what exercises to help you achieve your objectives.

An important step before you change what you eat for every meal is to see how you eat.

You're only able to eat once or twice a day.

You only eat once a day, but the meal is high in calories.

You consume three healthy foods per day but prefer to cheat between meals that are high in calories and fat with unhealthy snacks?

The critical issue is, to be honest with yourself in order to take the necessary steps to change the way you eat in order to improve your progress with weight loss and good health.

If you have honestly looked at how you eat, commit yourself to eat 5-6 small meals a day. This will improve your appetite for constant fat burning and the calories you eat. That idea should not cause a sudden panic, because you probably eat a comparable number of times a day if you truly take all of the treats consumed all day long into account. We change something that you are already doing to make it safer to increase your metabolic rate for better fat burning.

Foods must be removed from the diet to lose weight and maintain health.

The first products that are removed or reduced by your diet should be the foods high in fat and fried. These fatty foods are stored in the fat stores of the body and prevent pounds and inches from being lost.

Reduce your intake of milk products with high-fat content, such as 1 percent or 2 percent milk.

Begin to eat high-protein foods like whey, sweet beef, chicken, fish, turkey, salmon, and eggs. Eating high-protein foods helps boost your metabolism and rebuild your muscle during your weight loss practice routine.

Fatty acids in fish are beneficial to a healthy diet and improve your bones, teeth, clots, and hair's strength.

Be careful to avoid snack foods with excessive fat or high calories. Eating fruit or vegetables for snacks is a healthy way to control your calorie consumption.

Foods, including nuts, seeds, and flax oil, are major sources of the essential fatty acids which your body has to work properly. You will continue to go towards your healthy weight loss goals when you eat nuts and seeds as a snack instead of chips or other bad snacks.

For good health and weight loss, drinking adequate water is important. Trying to drink at least eight eighteen ounce glasses of water a day will keep you hydrated and full, making the appetite for high-calorie and fatty snacks unhealthy less likely. Adequate hydration of body cells and organs is important for the proper functioning and the disposal of waste products of the bodies.

Including a healthy multivitamin to your diet will help replace the nutrients that you might lack because of your past dietary habits.

We all want results now in this fast-paced world of multiple tasks. Procrastinating with weight loss and better health can cause frustration or chronic medical problems such as heart disease, diabetes, high blood pressure, strokes, and death.

Trying to lose 10-20 pounds for a short time and keep it away also contributes to unhealthy habits and disappointment as you regain all the weight you have lost. The time is not very good when you lose a considerable amount of weight every time you eat, but at the end of the year, you still weigh the same thing.

Depending on your current weight, you may lose this year 52 pounds rather than the yo yo-yo effect during previous weight loss attempts.

It doesn't matter whether you're morbidly odious or just want to drop a few pounds to the beach or wedding a friend, start taking a step back right now, take a deep breath and concentrate on studying, knowing, and using a simple solution to lose a pound a week.

Your progress each week improves your self-esteem and motivates you to maintain this simple weight loss diet and exercise, which will make you look sexier and healthier for years to come.

CONCLUSION

To keep overweight or obese people fat away and to keep them safe and productive for life, this stimulates the body to release stored fat and to use it for energy. A program of fat loss is distinct from a program of weight loss. The system works with your body and does not work against it to optimize the ability of your body to lose fat. The waistline, knees, buttocks, and upper arms you want to lose fat. You don't want to lose the density of muscle, water, or bone.

Popular diets for weight loss are a dangerous path. Many common diets require high amounts of protein food, for example, but excess protein causes stress on kidneys and stones because you can't digest the protein properly. It should also be noted that low-calorie diets do not improve diabetes or cardiac conditions as fat loss is inefficient. In fact, the body draws from the protein if it drops in caloric intake and is not selective where it derives from, including the heart and kidneys.

A glycemic diet is key to a healthy body that is lean. You can control what is put into your body and regulate blood sugar levels from a chemical perspective is the most effective way to release your fat burning capacity. You can control the dramatic growth of blood sugar, which pose serious threats to your health by taking a low glycemic diet.

The Glycemic Index (GI) is the new healthy eating norm. It was recently published by Harvard University Medical School in a new food pyramid. GI is the indicator of how much the blood sugar and insulin response in a particular food increase. The GI is the rate at which the blood sugar rises after you feed. A high glycemic load raises your blood sugar rapidly, causing insulin to rise and locking your fat. Also, non-fat foods will quickly become fat if insulin response is activated. We want the fat to be burned for energy. Low glycemic intake works with your body to prevent the insulin from spreading and to release stored fat for energy.

It is easy to change to a low GI diet because it is not difficult to calculate or continually focus on low fat or calories. You just have to replace your high GI food with low GI foods. If, as a country, we pay more attention to our diet and choose our food based on the use of low glycemic foods, the incidence of diabetes and obesity will decline dramatically.

Physical activity is a requirement of any plan for good health. Operation lights up the burning fat furnace. Any workout or exercise plan will begin with light to moderate effort and gradually increase the level of activity over time. Get off the stairs, or walk-all this enhances our physical activity. Start slowly, but start. Know the limits and do not push beyond.

Most people look at dietary pills that actually deplete the body of nutrients that can affect the normal function of the metabolism. We, therefore, need nutrients in the form of supplements for the normal functioning of metabolism. Supplements are used to balance the nutrients available in the body.

You need multivitamins and minerals in a nutrient matrix that is specifically designed to support the ability of your body to use fat. A supplement that provides important nutrients for antioxidants and stress. The bodies do not have over 400 toxins 40 years ago, most of which are contained, infant. When you begin to break this fat down, it releases these toxins. If the body doesn't have enough antioxidants help, metabolism slows down. This is a common cause of the plateau with most weight schemes. An antioxidant-rich in vitamins also improves blood glucose levels, bone health, liver, and nervous system.

You may need to raise your metabolic rate to optimize the capacity of your body to burn fat in the most effective fat loss programs. Once again, a healthy natural product that provides energy and improves your metabolic rate and regulates sugar in the blood and reduces appetite is required. The drug would give the problems caused by many appetite control items, a feeling of strength, and vitality. It shouldn't cause the jitters, for example.

For wellbeing and weight reduction, a high fiber diet is ideal. A fiber product is often required for a sense of fullness and for the health benefits of the digestion and colon. The fiber complex will spread softly in your stomach to create a sense of completeness. Fiber also leads to the elimination of food cravings.

Most plans for weight loss include a substitute food drink. Ensure that your meal replacement drink is low in glycemia and provides the nutrients that your body needs to feel full and delicious. The goal is to provide nutrition for the busy lifestyles of today.

Water is one of our diet's most important nutrients. Many adults need 8-10 glasses of water per day. Without enough water, you can not extract toxins. Drink a glass of water half an hour prior to a meal to prevent excessive intake and hydration. Just make sure you drink enough water before, during, and after workouts. Drinking the right amount of water will give you significant benefits and speed up the loss of weight.

Lightning Source UK Ltd.
Milton Keynes UK
UKHW022026150121
377139UK00003B/243